THE
essential
fertility
GUIDE

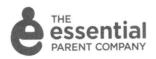

THE
essential
PARENT COMPANY

Professor Robert Winston

D0529250

Publishing Director Sarah Lavelle
Commissioning Editor Lisa Pendreigh
Project Editor Victoria Marshallsay
Creative Director Helen Lewis
Designer Emily Lapworth
Production Director Vincent Smith
Production Controller Tom Moore

First published in 2015 by
Quadrille Publishing

Quadrille is an imprint of Hardie Grant
www.hardiegrant.com.au

Quadrille Publishing, Pentagon House
52–54 Southwark Street, London SE1 1UN
www.quadrille.co.uk

Cataloguing in Publication Data:
a catalogue record for this book
is available from the British Library.

ISBN: 978 184949 540 0

Printed in China

10 9 8 7 6 5 4 3 2 1

Introduction
By Professor Robert Winston

I have had the most privileged professional life. I have worked with so many people who have had difficulty getting pregnant. They tolerated my frequent failures rather than my clinic's sporadic success. They taught me a great deal; I owe a huge debt to numbers of patients who persuaded me to listen, opening my eyes to their sadness, and my scant understanding of it. They were experiencing a void in one crucial area of human existence. Having a child is the most life-enhancing and life-changing experience. When I consider my own scientific and other meagre successes, I know only too well that having the privilege of nurturing my own children has genuinely been the most important achievement. I never faced their personal void.

This handbook is an attempt to help those people who find that they are having difficulty conceiving. It is not a complete treatise on every aspect of infertility, its causes or its treatment, nor is it meant to cover every aspect of in vitro fertilisation (IVF) and all advanced fertility treatments. But I have written it in an attempt to help people to ask their doctors the right questions and, where needed, to understand their treatment. The causes of infertility are very complex – much more so than is generally recognised. Treatments like IVF are difficult and demanding, as well as expensive. They are also a lottery – often there is not much rhyme nor reason why one couple succeeds and others don't. Or why some patients never conceive when nothing appears to be wrong, while others get pregnant apparently against all odds.

IVF is now very widely used – indeed, in my view, far too often. Yet IVF is seen to be the standard fertility treatment. People reading this book will realise that there are many different reasons why a couple may be having difficulty conceiving. Above all, I hope they will see that making a diagnosis before treatment and using a specific, often cheaper, treatment is often more satisfactory.

I am also aware that the government's own regulatory authority, the Human Fertilisation and Embryology Authority (HFEA) does not do a great job in preventing the financial exploitation of patients. Nor does it always explain infertility treatment well. To make matters worse, the NHS is not nearly interested enough in infertility – it frequently does not recognise the real pain and great sadness this symptom causes. Regrettably some doctors in the NHS do not take infertility sufficiently seriously to gain expertise in its management or to answer patients' questions in enough detail.

There are few places where prospective patients can get totally unbiased and independent information that is accurate. This handbook is an attempt at addressing this. Readers may know that I am Chairman of Genesis Research Trust, which funds what we regard to be the most advanced research into women's health. In our laboratories research into both male and female infertility has also been carried out for some years. The Trust runs a website www.genesisresearchtrust.com where we try to answer infertile patients' queries without bias. From time to time, whenever, for example, there is an announcement of a new development or a query about a particular treatment, we give independent advice. I have now retired from practice and none of us at Genesis runs a clinic – nor do we treat patients – so we have little conflict of interests. But we suggest that people logging onto our website may care to give a donation if they wish, but we do not check on this. Sometimes giving such advice is complicated and time-consuming and often we need to trawl the latest research to ensure the accuracy of what we write. Any donations are pooled to help research into the treatments we think will be important in the future.

Chapter 1: The experience of infertility

I would like to begin this book with a short chapter about what the experience of infertility often means. As I said previously, I've been lucky: I have never had this problem. You might feel that my observations, gained from nearly 40 years clinical work talking and listening to many couples, may be flawed or inaccurate. If so, I apologise and am prepared to understand the objections of those who know better from first-hand experience.

In the UK, we boast that the British invention of in vitro fertilisation (IVF) is one of the ten most important scientific advances of the last 50 years. But it is cruel irony that most people in this country who might benefit from it are excluded. We know from quite good statistics that approximately one in every seven couples in the UK experience some difficulty in conception. Yet in 2014, more than 35 years after the birth of the first test tube baby, only about 47,000 women were treated by IVF throughout the UK. And some of these were unquestionably foreign nationals coming here for private treatment. The annual growth in the number of IVF cycles in Britain is miserable. We treat only 10 per cent of those couples who could be helped. Even if you are lucky enough to get free IVF, the NHS limits the number of treatment cycles you can have – giving most patients no more than a 25 per cent chance of success. The government's National Institute for Health and Care Excellence (NICE), has recommended three treatment cycles for those needing this treatment, but the NHS frequently limits each patient to one cycle, a cruelly inadequate decision. What other NHS treatment would be abandoned less than halfway through its justified course? Thereafter, you are on your own. If you want a reasonable chance of a baby, you will need to pay high fees for private treatment. Moreover, in many parts of the UK, a postcode lottery exists with no NHS treatment.

And records show that there are around 920,000 pregnancies each year in the UK but only 750,000 births. Many pregnancies end in miscarriage, a loss of life causing grief, depression and mourning, and in the vast majority no serious attempt is made to ascertain the cause. The apparent attitude of many doctors and nurses, and certainly most hospitals, is that miscarriages are so common that they are not worth worrying about – it's simple for couples to try again.

Early in my career it became apparent that there were many individuals whose predicament was not taken seriously by their friends, family, our society, or my profession. Indeed, when I was first offered the post of Director of the Fertility Clinic at Hammersmith Hospital, to follow Professor John McClure Browne who had established it, a very senior consultant said to me, 'Why do you want to work in the Futility Clinic?' These attitudes were common amongst colleagues who should have known better. If it hadn't been for Professor McClure Browne's support and encouragement, and his compassion, I would never have entered this rewarding speciality and this book is dedicated to his memory.

The urge to reproduce is deeply burnt into human consciousness. The desire is not merely the hedonism of a sexual encounter, though that is powerful enough and part of the process. It is innate, instinctual, essentially programmed through evolution. When we look at our own offspring, that genetic imperative seems obvious. Babies are noisy, smelly, highly inconvenient, cause sleeplessness, destroy free time and are extremely expensive. Yet we feel like melting when we see them. This is not rational – it is in our genes.

How does it feel to be infertile? How does it affect your self-esteem? How do you cope with friendships and social contacts? How do you protect yourself against repeated disappointments and intrusive treatments? How do you protect your relationship with your partner? How do you decide when to call an end to treatment? These are all questions I attempt to answer throughout this book.

How do people react to infertility?

Of course, one person's experience of infertility may vary greatly from another's. Some are not much disturbed; but most couples go through strong emotions and their feelings tend to form a pattern.

Initial anxiety

Most people are not terribly worried if they don't conceive in the first few months. Older women may feel time is running out and may become concerned sooner. For others, the growing realisation of a problem is often shrugged off at first. It is more common for the female partner to take the initiative in seeking help. Occasionally this is without her partner's knowledge. Men may seem unconcerned or indifferent, yet usually mask a gnawing doubt. I have known some couples that have worried for years without seeking medical advice. For others, the arrival of the next menstrual period is a moment of crisis every month. Worse still is a negative pregnancy test after a delay in the arrival of an expected period.

Disbelief

The first real shock of infertility often comes when a couple see friends starting a family. The reality of their own situation is hard to believe and one or other partner might deny any responsibility for their problem. Just before writing this book I was talking to Angela, a friend who had been very distressed – she had gone through numerous negative tests but assumed she must be responsible for her failure to conceive. Her husband, Paul, repeatedly denied that he might have a problem, because, unknown to Angela, a girlfriend of his had had a miscarriage nine years previously. Only after Angela had persisted with numerous tests – including laparoscopy and staying overnight in hospital – did Paul hesitantly go to a doctor, who was in turn rather unhelpful and dismissive. Eventually Paul had two semen tests. Even when the tests were abnormal, he did not accept he needed treatment. Eventually the marriage broke up. There may, for all I know, have been many reasons for their separation, but on talking to Angela I had no doubt that the pressure of infertility played a major part. Angela, at 42, had a baby, having conceived naturally with a new husband. Paul's story shows that anxiety and fear, as well as denial, are common. These emotions can corrode a relationship. Paul's experience, which Angela deeply regretted, shows that the first visit to a specialist can be much more traumatic than many doctors realise.

Anger, guilt and frustration

Infertility produces bursts of anger, sometimes directed towards one's spouse, the doctor, the clinic, or tests giving dubious results. Couples can feel most frustrated when a complicated test like laparoscopy (see page 42) fails to find an abnormality. Discovering that something is definitely wrong may mean that the chances of a pregnancy are not good, but some people are more frustrated if the laparoscopic findings are normal. People also direct anger at themselves. Anger with a partner is common, especially when that person feels disinclined to have tests, or take their partner's distress seriously.

Feelings of guilt occur frequently. The idea you brought your infertility upon yourself is often experienced at some stage, which is why I have always been reluctant to suggest to a man or a woman that blockage of the fine pipes in the testis or the Fallopian tubes might be due to some past infection. Some fertility clinics place great emphasis on testing for chlamydia; it is claimed the bacteria are a common cause of blocked Fallopian tubes after sexually transmitted infection. To my mind this relationship is poorly established. Doctors should not increase the guilt feelings of people with pelvic inflammatory disease who think they damaged themselves.

Couples may also resent that others do not understand how they feel or be bitterly unhappy at losing control – at having to rely on a doctor to help with what should happen naturally. Anger may be felt, too, with people who have children, or waiting in a clinic where there may be women attending for antenatal appointments or those requesting termination of a pregnancy.

Depression and feelings of pointlessness

Nearly all infertile people experience sadness at some stage. It develops gradually and may become most acute just before or just after your period, especially if it is delayed.

You may just feel tearful. But periods of sleeplessness, loss of appetite, or disturbances such as headaches, loss of energy and constipation, are common. Sometimes this becomes so great that periods are irregular, which adds to the anxiety. Feeling that things are not worth enjoying, or it is not worth trying to be successful in your job – because you have no children to appreciate your material advantages are frequent. You may come to think that there is no point in going to normal social engagements or parties. Depression can lead people to withdraw, avoid friendships and refuse to share their feelings. Isolation is common and it often comes as a surprise to infertile couples that others have exactly the same feelings. Infertility may be a symptom shared by many, but childless couples often think they are alone.

Loss of self-esteem can cause both partners to feel like failures. For a man, infertility may first present as a problem just when he is trying hard to develop a career. If his job is going badly, he may feel particularly worthless, as if he is a 'double failure'. Either partner may feel that they have let their other half down and find that more distressing.

Problems with sex

Many couples find their sexual relationship is affected at some stage. Lovemaking loses spontaneity, becoming planned and cold. Pleasure may become a thing of the past and some women stop having orgasms. Men may experience impotence or premature ejaculation – both of which, of course, make conception more difficult. Very often, the need to have sex produces anxiety. So many women say, 'there seems to be no point in sex anymore – my body can't respond and is just useless'.

Monica is typical of many patients I treated. This vibrant, fun-loving extrovert, told me that after five years of trying to conceive, having sex, 'makes me feel like an empty vessel'. It is common, too, for people to feel unattractive or unloved, so many find they have sex at increasingly infrequent intervals. Unfortunately, some doctors show little understanding and their advice to have intercourse at 'precisely the right time' can make matters seem worse.

When sex stops being enjoyable, this itself may increase difficulties in conceiving; some specialists believe loss of female orgasm could decrease fertility. Whether pleasurable intercourse improves the chance of conception is not clear, but it might be better for you to have sex when you really feel like it, even though you think you may be missing the time around ovulation. One or two nights of pleasure may be better than daily attempts at frustration.

Desperation

Such feelings frequently lead to desperation, particularly amongst women, who may feel the burden more acutely. So many fix their idea on one particular treatment resolutely believing it will solve the problem. A common idea is that IVF will be the solution irrespective of the cause of the infertility. Couples peruse the success rates announced by various clinics and any published by the Human Fertilisation and Embryology Authority (HFEA). But simply because one IVF clinic is advertising a greater success rate than another means little when it comes to your own treatment. As with any medical condition, the cause of the infertility is most critical, and success varies accordingly. Some clinics have substantially better success rates because of the clientele they treat. For example, a condition causing 'mild' infertility – such as failure of regular ovulation – will be easier to treat than tubal disease.

Despair causes people to chase a host of different, unproven therapies. These include acupuncture, aromatherapy, reflexology, psychotherapy, herbal medicine, Chinese treatments, vitamin supplements and homeopathy. None of these is likely to be of the slightest benefit in normally nourished individuals.

Grief and bereavement

Persistent infertility causes grief. Feeling hopeless can lead to obsession, the desire to chase every possible treatment, no matter how illogical. Grieving couples frequently seek repeated medical opinions when an earlier one seems unsatisfactory.

Grief can be a reaction to the inability to give life. The loss of a parent or a friend is usually supported by others, but infertile couples often feel that they have no one to turn to for support. Their parents may refuse to accept the situation and it can be very difficult to explain how you feel. Friends who have children may appear embarrassed or unfeeling at the anger and frustration you live with every day.

Grief can eventually be positive. If you are absolutely infertile, the natural process of grief, bereavement and mourning may lead to a final healing. This can resolve an otherwise entirely destructive situation.

Can infertility be psychological?

At some stage many infertile couples wonder whether their tangled emotions are causing infertility. If you have been trying for a long time with no obvious cause for your childlessness, you may well think your anxiety itself is the problem.

That vicious circle is one difficulty; the harder and longer you try to conceive, the more disturbed you feel. Your specialist may encourage you to get out of your domestic environment a bit more. Weekends away, short holidays, even an afternoon's walk together in a pleasant park nearby, may be invaluable if things are getting on top of you. Relaxing together regularly may help break any tension and allow better communication. It may help improve any difficulty with sex and other pent-up thoughts. Some women find giving up their job has been most therapeutic and others, unsurprisingly, that starting a new job is a great benefit.

The evidence for one's emotional state being a major cause for infertility is sketchy. It might contribute, but only to a tiny degree. Being aware of this problem and meeting it sensibly can be important, not only to improve your chances, but also to help over the long periods of uncertainty.

The case against 'psychological' infertility

If it were true that emotional turmoil is an important cause of infertility, people under exceptional stress would not get pregnant. This does not seem to be the case. Take the common example of a young woman having sex with her boyfriend and not using contraception. She may be desperately worried that she might get pregnant, so much so that it causes enormous stress in her relationship. This never seems to reduce the disasters that we see, and frightened requests for secret abortions. Another example is women who suffer the shocking trauma of rape, with its horrific stress. Yet statistics show that the chances of getting pregnant after a single act of rape are actually often higher than the chances of conceiving at other times. Why this happens is unclear, but it doesn't support the idea that infertility is caused by extreme stress. If stress were a serious bar to conception, you would not expect women suffering great hardship to conceive readily. Yet unwanted pregnancy is very common where the most severe privation is common – psychological infertility doesn't seem a problem in famine-struck Asia or Eritrea. Finally, think of couples undergoing IVF: by the time an embryo is transferred, there is often severe stress. Research suggests that their attitude and emotional state has remarkably little effect on the chances of conception.

The case for 'psychological' infertility
There is, of course, limited evidence for emotionally-induced infertility. Many animals in zoos, even when well fed and well treated, are less fertile than when they are in the wild. Zoos worldwide have always had difficulty, for example, trying to breed giant pandas. Cows whose routine is disturbed may have a lower milk yield and may not come into calf. Most research workers know that one of the most fertile creatures, the rabbit, breeds with difficulty if there is much stress in the premises where they are kept. I remember the difficulties we had in our own animal house when a new technician, Brian, was first employed to look after my rabbits. One morning I found out he used to come into the room that contained their hutches loudly singing hymns – 'Onward Christian Soldiers' was a favourite. They started to breed again only when he made much less noise and they got used to him. I often wondered whether they would have been more fertile had he sung 'Jerusalem' with its green fields.

Some humans may react to stress equally badly. It is well documented that women in prison often suffer irregular periods. Women who were brutally kept in concentration camps during the Nazi regime often had severe disturbances of menstruation and probably did not ovulate.

Perhaps one of the most often quoted examples of 'psychological' infertility regards couples who, after years of trying hard for a baby, finally adopt. Within weeks of the adoption, they conceive naturally without medical help. It is difficult to say whether this is just chance. Ellen and Paul tried for a baby for six years. Extensive tests gave no obvious cause for infertility. Ellen had never had children, though Paul had had a child by another woman years earlier. In spite of this, Paul's tests were not entirely normal and I thought it was quite likely that the cause of the problem lay with him. I continued to treat them both, but five long years continued without pregnancy. One day Ellen came to see me by herself. This was in the days before intracytoplasmic sperm injection (see ICSI, page 106) and we both felt depressed that she might just have to accept Paul's slightly low sperm count. Then Ellen broke down and said she had been hiding something. She was sure the problem was hers, she told me, because for three years she been also trying to get pregnant by a boyfriend, Simon. Simon was married with three young children and Paul knew nothing of this relationship.

'It must be my fault but how can I reassure Paul who feels so guilty,' she said.

I saw a very unhappy Ellen for six more months. At the back of my mind I felt that she ought to resolve her trouble by making a definite break; we had discussed various possibilities, including separation and possibly divorce. She told me she desperately wanted to marry Simon and he had told her he would leave his family. One day Ellen attended my clinic, deeply upset:

'It's over. Simon and his wife are emigrating. He's going to work in California and I've told Paul everything. Now I'll never have a baby.'

I gently suggested perhaps this was for the best. Seven weeks later Ellen returned to my clinic with a positive pregnancy test, undoubtedly with Paul's child. Such stories are not that unusual in fertility clinics.

The speed that people get pregnant when an emotional situation like Ellen's is resolved makes me wonder that, after all, we sometimes cause our own problems.

Other pressures on infertile couples

Parents can make life awkward for some couples. They may show considerable sympathy when they learn you are having difficulties, but they may feel deprived by the thought that there will be no grandchildren. They may put you under unspoken pressure by never raising the subject; or they may pressurise you by suggesting what you should do, or where you should go for treatment, even though you have made certain decisions. Occasionally, there can be a hint of criticism. In some families, your parents-in-law may give you the feeling that they think it is your fault, even if the cause is unknown. An infertile woman may begin to believe that her parents-in-law view her as an inadequate spouse.

Sometimes a sibling may have presented your parents or parents-in-law with grandchildren and their affection for them, or their pleasure at a new pregnancy, can be particularly painful. Sisters can be a threat, too, and it is remarkably common for infertile women to find it impossible to spend time in a brother or sister's house, especially if it is full of young children.

Another pressure may be the attitude of friends. Even your closest friends may try to protect you by refusing to bring up the subject of children. This reinforces the guilt and inadequacy you feel about being infertile. Although you feel unable to mention the subject yourself, the conspiracy of silence increases your lack of self-esteem. A dinner party with people you know slightly may be a hardship. It is surprising how often the subject of children crops up followed by stifled embarrassment from those who simply wish to protect you.

Miscarriage and ectopic pregnancy

Miscarriage is extremely common; one in four of all pregnancies miscarry in the first four months of pregnancy, usually before the tenth week. A later chapter deals with miscarriage but it is important to understand that infertile couples are more prone to miscarriages and they are increasingly common by the time a woman reaches the age of 42. It is particularly hard to be trying a long time for a pregnancy, find exultantly that you are pregnant, and then have that frightening show of blood and then that lost life. Our society does not take miscarriages very seriously (we don't have funerals for tiny embryos a few millimetres long), but an infertile couple can find it devastating. Many women who have had miscarriages remember that dreaded date each subsequent year and mourn that loss.

Most miscarriages are completely unexplained and often the medical profession does little to establish the cause. So often a woman will be told by her GP or a junior hospital doctor 'Well, in a few weeks you will be ready to start again', without acknowledging the anguish. Moreover, there is usually not much treatment once a miscarriage is underway – most of them cannot be stopped once the bleeding has started unless it is slight. The trauma of a hospital admission for a 'scrape' is also unsettling – particularly (as is generally the case) there can be a long wait to get the operation to have the uterus 'cleaned'. Moreover, patients with miscarriages may be on wards with women having abortions or those with serious illnesses. Ward staff may forget the feelings of women who are undergoing a miscarriage; as it happens so frequently, it is seen as rather trivial. Ectopic pregnancy is even more emotionally fraught. Not only is the loss of an embryo very disturbing, but because an ectopic pregnancy is potentially life-threatening due to internal bleeding, it may cause fear. This anxiety may continue long after emergency treatment. Woman who have had one ectopic pregnancy are more likely to have another. Some women get so worried about this that they may avoid getting pregnant again even though a baby is deeply desired.

Chapter 2: The causes of infertility

Throughout this book I repeatedly assert one thing: the best chance for successful fertility treatment is to do everything reasonable to find out the basic cause of your infertility. The emphasis these days is heavily on in vitro fertilisation (IVF), so couples need to know as much about their situation as possible to ask the right questions and have some proper control over their treatment.

Understanding infertility

It is really important to understand that infertility is merely a symptom that something is wrong. It is not a disease, but usually the result of a disease process. There are numerous causes and the best treatment may be different in each circumstance. Unfortunately, the massive publicity given to IVF has led to most people believing that it is almost the only treatment and the most successful. This is utterly wrong.

Couples rush into IVF far too frequently. There are so many freestanding IVF clinics nowadays that there is a real chance of being referred to a clinic without the competence or interest in offering anything other than IVF. Regrettably, in the commercial sector, where most IVF is done because NHS provision is so inadequate, the pressure for the clinic to offer profitable IVF rather than another treatment is strong. Of course, there are ethical private practitioners. But it is easier to feed patients into a standard system, a mechanised process such as IVF, rather than spend sufficient time investigating the underlying cause. IVF practice is immensely profitable, and regrettably in some centres there is a risk of it being offered even when it may not be the most suitable treatment.

As with all medical conditions, merely treating the symptom alone is seldom good medicine. Let me explain. If you went to your GP complaining of chest pain, you would consider him a very bad doctor if he immediately referred you for heart surgery. If your pain is due to bronchitis, an antibiotic is required, chest pain can be caused by indigestion so antacids are best, or you could merely have a bruise or a strained chest muscle, or possibly a broken rib – in which case pain-relief may be needed. On rare occasions, you could be suffering from a cancer of the oesophagus. None of these conditions necessitates heart surgery.

Very roughly, failure to conceive is caused by a female problem in just over a third of cases. In about one third, the problem is that the man is sub-fertile, and in the remainder both partners are responsible. In addition, a substantial number of couples will have what is referred to as 'unexplained infertility'. But often more detailed testing unveils a probable cause.

It is frequently said that infertility is on the increase, but there is less evidence for this. It is probably due to women leaving childbearing until later in life. In advanced countries most women now gain education, experience and skills before trying for a baby, but as a woman grows older natural fertility declines. Undoubtedly more women in their late thirties or early forties now seek treatment.

What are some of the more likely causes?

You may be surprised how many causes of infertility there are and how the best treatment generally depends on treating the cause.

Female infertility

In the UK, the most common cause of female infertility is failure to ovulate (around 30 per cent). Damage to the Fallopian tubes is less frequent (about 25 per cent of cases). Endometriosis (see page 130) is found in perhaps 20 per cent of infertile women, but usually does not cause infertility (this mostly depends on the amount of scarring and whether the ovaries are involved). Abnormalities of the uterus are quite common, but my experience suggests these are not always discovered by many of the routine tests. Reduced ovarian reserve is more common now because women are trying to have a baby later in life.

Multiple causes

Many couples have two, or occasionally more, causes for difficulties in conception. In the large London teaching hospital where I worked, about 12–15 per cent of patients had multiple causes. For example, a woman may suffer from mild tubal disease as well as intermittent failure to ovulate. Or, a sub-fertile woman may be married to a man with a lowered sperm count. In general couples with multiple causes are particularly suitable for IVF.

In about 20 per cent of couples, the only abnormal finding is a poor sperm count, in another 25 per cent it is a major contributory cause. Occasionally, there may be male infertility even when the sperm look microscopically normal. Problems with sex or difficulty with ejaculation possibly account for around 3 per cent of all infertility.

Unexplained infertility

So-called unexplained infertility seems to vary greatly. Some surveys suggest that this may account for around 20–25 per cent of infertility, but this estimate may depend on the extent of detailed testing. At Hammersmith Hospital, with a policy of exhaustive testing, around 10 per cent of patients could be said to have unexplained infertility. Recently, correspondence with professionals who treat women from strictly orthodox Jewish communities in London suggests that the incidence of 'unexplained infertility' amongst them is no more than 2–5 per cent. This may be related to pelvic infection as this is uncommon in these women, perhaps because usually they have only one sexual partner. Some people with a diagnosis of so-called unexplained infertility have often had pelvic inflammatory disease in the past, but unless a telescope inspection of the pelvis is carried out (see laparoscopy, page 42) the scarring left by infection may not be identified. Unfortunately, laparoscopy is now less frequently done under the NHS than it should be. NICE has recommended, with dubious wisdom, limited indications for using it. As a result, doctors feel they should avoid it unless they are strongly convinced of its necessity. Ironically, this 'cost-saving' approach results in more patients having expensive IVF treatment than necessary.

Sometimes a diagnosis made with hindsight, after treatment, perhaps with IVF. Once an IVF cycle is completed, we find obscure causes for failure to conceive. For example, very occasionally there may be no fertilisation even when there is a normal sperm count. This suggests a problem with the sperm, or occasionally the egg, not revealed by routine tests. Possibly a genetic or molecular reason for this failure is only revealed by IVF.

SYMPTOMS ASSOCIATED WITH FEMALE INFERTILITY

Symptom or history	Result or possible cause
Absent periods	Probably not ovulating; damage to lining of uterus; genetic problem of some kind; anorexia or response to vigorous exercise particularly if underweight; various hormone disorders; premature menopause.
Very infrequent or irregular periods	Likely to be not ovulating regularly; possible loss of ovarian reserve.
Recent increasingly painful periods	Endometriosis or adenomyosis; polyp in the uterus; fibroids; inflammation or pelvic inflammatory disease.
Increasingly heavy periods	Fibroids; hormonal disorder of some kind; premenopausal.
Increasing weight gain	Polycystic ovaries; not ovulating.

Increasing hair growth	Polycystic ovary syndrome; ovarian tumour; adrenal disease.
Bleeding between periods	Endometriosis or adenomyosis; hormonal problem; uterine polyp.
Previous operation on the cervix for abnormal smear	Abnormalities of sperm entry into the uterus.
Previous operation for ovarian cyst	Adhesions between tubes and ovaries; ovarian failure.
Previous peritonitis or appendicitis	Adhesions or blocked Fallopian tubes.
Problems with contraceptive coil requiring removal	Damage to tubes or adhesions in the uterus.
Infection after birth or complicated labour	Pelvic adhesions or blocked tubes.
Recurrent miscarriages	Uterus not anatomically normal; chromosomal or genetic problem; haematological or immune disorder.
Previous ectopic pregnancy	Undiagnosed problem in the opposite tube.
Vaginal discharge	Vaginal or cervical infection; hydrosalpinx; fibroid polyp; adenomyosis; uterine tumour.

SYMPTOMS ASSOCIATED WITH MALE INFERTILITY

Symptom or history	Result or possible cause
Mumps especially during adult or adolescent life	Arrest of sperm development.
Old testicle injury, perhaps sport or twisted testicle	Poor seminal quality; absent sperm.
Previous undescended testicle	Poor sperm count motility.
Previous hernia operation	Low sperm count.
Past inflammation or cyst of testes	Low sperm count.
Inflammation of prostate gland	Seminal infection; white cells.
Operations on bladder or prostate	Impotence.
Heavy smoking or alcohol/drug usage	Impotence; poor sperm count.
Orgasm without release of seminal fluid	Sperm in urine.
Previous sexual infection, e.g. gonorrhoea	Poor sperm count or motility; blocked tubules or vas.

History of cystic fibrosis	Blockage of vas deferens.
Testicular swelling	Blockage of vas deferens; hydrocoele.
Small testes	Poor count or no sperm.
Testicular malignancy	Poor count or no sperm.
Certain prescription drugs; anti-cancer drugs; methotrexate; sulfasalazine; some herbal remedies; anabolic steroids	All reduced sperm counts.
Occupational: possibly long distance drivers, steel workers, deep-sea divers, exposure to mercury, lead, cadmium or pesticides	All reduced sperm counts.
Obesity	Reduced sperm counts.

Choosing treatment

Each condition causing infertility may require different treatment. Yet, increasingly, women with a simple problem such as failure to ovulate are immediately offered IVF. Do not forget, no matter what individual clinics may advertise, IVF is actually successful in only about 25 per cent of cycles. In the USA, the results seem slightly better. Having worked extensively in the American system and seen it at first hand, I can assure you this does not mean that doctors and clinics there are more skilful. The method of reporting their results may introduce a bias which is unacceptable in Europe. Of course, though each cycle of IVF may only have a one in four chance of success, it can be repeated. But neither the NHS nor most people's finances will allow many repeated attempts. After the third attempt, IVF success rates tend to decrease, a good reason to try and ascertain the underlying cause of the infertility. Apart from having spent a huge amount of money and experienced considerable stress, it often proves difficult to return to simpler treatments after IVF. There is always the temptation to try another IVF cycle with a slightly different recipe. Sometimes the underlying cause of the infertility, possibly undiagnosed, will have prevented IVF from working at all. Marjorie, a 35-year-old patient at Hammersmith, had had a miscarriage six months after she married. Because she was infertile she was referred to a fertility clinic in the Midlands where she was inadequately investigated and had seven treatment cycles. In all she spent £33,600. Each cycle produced eggs that were fertilised and with each treatment, fresh or frozen embryos were transferred to her uterus. Each time she had the increasingly devastating news of a failed pregnancy test. The clinic offered her an eighth cycle, but she decided on a second opinion. Only when she was investigated using a simple X-ray (see HSG, page 40) costing £250, were adhesions in her uterus identified. A simple 10-minute operation resulted in their removal and she then became pregnant without further treatment. Her first baby, a girl, was born 14 months later. She now has three children, each spaced almost two years apart. I get a Christmas photograph from her every year.

Finally, an important reason for making a diagnosis is that most people who fail to get pregnant find they gain considerable comfort from knowing what is wrong. Sometimes they find it easier to come to terms with their situation because they feel they understand things better.

Chapter 3: Making a diagnosis

One thing is obvious – and should be clear after reading the beginning of this book – please do not start having tests after you have commenced treatment. Do not go for IVF treatment without a clear idea about why you need it. Most infertile couples do not require this complex treatment.

Humans are amongst the most naturally infertile mammals on the planet. The overall monthly chance of a normal woman getting pregnant is no more than about 18–25 per cent per menstrual cycle. Humans are only fertile for about one-third of their life, becoming less so with age. We spend a long time growing to maturity and a depressingly longer time as menopausal adults.

Most couples take an average of five months to conceive, and it really is not unusual to take longer. Testing is generally indicated after one year of childlessness unless there are specific indications that there may be a problem. Then earlier medical advice is justified. Symptoms indicating earlier investigation include very irregular or no periods, excessive hair growth, a history of abdominal surgery or a burst appendix, repeated miscarriage or an ectopic pregnancy, problems whilst wearing an intrauterine contraceptive coil, or a family history of early menopause. Men and women who have suffered genital tract infection may wish to seek earlier investigation, as should men with a swelling in the testis, a history of significant groin injury or testicular surgery. In particular, women over 30 years old are slightly less fertile and may take longer to get pregnant. Consequently, although there may be little wrong, they may wish to be investigated sooner.

What tests are important?

Once you seek help, a diagnosis may take six months. This may seem like a long time, but tests need to be coordinated with the menstrual cycle and it is most important that a thorough range of tests be carried out. Often a cause for the infertility is found halfway through testing and treatment can be started. Not infrequently there may well be more than one cause of infertility and a premature or incomplete diagnosis can lead to delaying effective treatment.

Make yourself as familiar with the various tests, which is another reason for writing this book – without knowledge it is difficult to know what questions you should ask. A good GP is invaluable at all stages as even experienced specialists can omit an important test and reminders can help. If you find asking difficult, discuss your case with your GP who will normally have made the original referral and should keep an eye on your care. Do not hesitate to say if you think tests are taking too long (or are not being done); he or she can speed up the process by writing to the consultant in charge. The specialist, whose practice depends on satisfying patients sent by GPs, will seldom take offence.

While GPs are generally in a position to organise some simple tests like a sperm count, most send their infertile patients to a specialist gynaecologist with experience in fertility medicine. If you have a particular clinic or specialist in mind, you can ask your GP to refer you accordingly. Nowadays, under the new NHS regulations, this is your right.

The first appointment

For the first hospital visit it is best if you attend with your partner. Hospitals and fertility clinics can be forbidding and it is good for morale to share what may be a stressful experience. The specialist will want to know how long you have been trying to conceive and about any previous pregnancies. Some women may naturally worry that they might be asked about a pregnancy of which their partner has no knowledge. If it is impossible to be candid during the joint visit, arrange to see the specialist alone on a separate occasion. Doctors will not reveal such private information to anyone else, including a partner.

The specialist should generally ask about any gynaecological history and the frequency of recent menstrual periods. He or she may also inquire about how often you both have sexual intercourse and whether you are experiencing any difficulties. Some couples may find such questions embarrassing, but they are obviously relevant.

The doctor should conduct an internal examination, although provided a woman is having regular intercourse and there is no history suggesting uterine abnormalities or an ovarian cyst, it may provide little information. If you are especially anxious this may be deferred until the next visit when confidence has been gained. It is an important examination as failure to diagnose a lump, such as a fibroid or an ovarian cyst, could have a bearing on treatment. Examination of men usually gives rather less information, even when there is an abnormal sperm count. But occasionally a damaged testis may be smaller than normal, or there may be cysts or abnormal swelling requiring special tests.

Tests for men

These range from assessing the number and quality of sperm, to hormone tests, ultrasound and chromosome evaluation.

Sperm counts

A full sperm assessment includes a range of measurements. A single normal sperm count does not necessarily indicate a man is fully fertile. Nor does one abnormal or low count necessarily mean that there is anything wrong. Nearly all men produce poor quality semen

TEST RESULTS

Most clinics will not generally give the results of sperm tests over the telephone. They will ensure whom they are talking to, and be able to provide proper emotional support if needed. It can be helpful, if possible, for both partners to go and get the test results together. It is an important time for both of them, and it can be a heavy burden for a woman to go to the clinic by herself to find that her partner has a possible problem.

occasionally, especially if they have had a recent illness or have been under stress. A man's fertility is assessed on the basis of several sperm counts and other sperm function tests.

Semen volume Following orgasm most men ejaculate around 2–5ml (a teaspoonful) of seminal fluid. If the volume is less, the man may not be producing enough secretions. However, producing semen for medical examination usually involves good juggling to get all the fluid collected in the ridiculously tiny pot that nearly all clinics provide. So it is quite common to miss some fluid from an ejaculate.

Sperm numbers Amazingly, there are normally more than 40 million in each millilitre of seminal fluid. One of the miracles of fertility is than an average man (if there is such a creature) produces around 200 million sperm in each ejaculate in just a teaspoon of fluid. Although it only takes one sperm to fertilise an egg, it seems almost unbelievable that there still may be a problem if there are fewer than 20 million in each millilitre. Many sperm are destroyed or lost inside the woman's body and others have abnormalities preventing fertilisation.

A count lower than 20 million per millilitre does not necessarily mean that a man is sterile. A few men are fully fertile even when they produce only two or three million sperm per millilitre. I met one man who only had one million sperm in his ejaculate, but he fathered three children with two different women before his current marriage. The wicked thought entered my suspicious mind that the children he claimed might not be his – but genetic testing on two confirmed his parentage. His third wife got pregnant shortly after these tests, but his sperm count never improved.

Sperm motility 40 per cent of the sperm should be moving. I've always been amazed when, looking down a microscope, how aimless most sperm are. Some move in circles, some zigzag, some look as if they are dithering and others as if they are having convulsions. The quality of movement is important; there are now sophisticated machines that can measure the speed of an individual sperm under the microscope and detect whether it is swimming in a straight line.

The shape and structure of a sperm A healthy sample usually contains around at least 65 per cent normal-looking sperm. Typical abnormalities include sperm with abnormal or double heads, or heads filled with rounded droplets. Sometimes defects in the middle of the sperm are seen, or spermatozoa with kinked and deformed tails. The significance of all these oddities is not fully understood but if there are a lot of abnormal sperm, it may mean that there is a testicular problem.

Viscosity of seminal fluid Some men produce very 'thick' seminal fluid. When first produced, fluid may be rather jelly-like, but it should liquefy. High viscosity may interfere with sperm motility. The significance of failure to liquefy is rather controversial because nobody knows what happens once the fluid is inside a woman's body. Nonetheless, it is regarded as a problem if the semen fails to liquefy in the open air within around two hours of its production; it may indicate a problem in the prostate gland or the sperm reservoirs inside the male genital tract.

Presence of clumping, bacteria, or white blood cells If sperm are stuck together this may indicate infection or possible antibodies to the sperm. The presence of many bacteria or white cells also indicates possible infection that may impair the sperm function.

Some laboratories culture the semen to identify any bacterium before antibiotic treatment. But cultures are unreliable unless the sperm are carefully collected. It is difficult to produce and ejaculate under sterile conditions, whilst holding that little pot.

Fructose levels If there are no sperm in the semen there may be a blockage above or below the seminal vesicles. These structures produce fructose, a form of sugar that is easily measured. If fructose is low, the blockage may be below the seminal vesicles. This information is obviously useful if a surgeon is planning to remove a blockage.

Presence of antibodies Antibodies are produced by our immune system in response to injury or infection, a vital part of the body's defences, When they attack the sperm they can impair function. The specialised tests for antibodies include the MAR (mixed antiglobulin reaction) test and the immune-bead test; the latter involves counting the proportion of sperm that stick to specially coated beads.

Split ejaculate test The first part of the ejaculate tends to be richer in sperm, even in men with low sperm counts. So a split ejaculate test can evaluate whether this 'concentrated' semen is worth collecting for artificial insemination. This investigation is now done infrequently as IVF is mostly used when the sperm count is low. Nonetheless it has a place, particularly for couples wishing to avoid IVF.

Tests for retrograde ejaculation Occasionally a man may have perfectly good sperm production, but the muscles that contract during orgasm do not function properly. This may be a problem in paraplegics, or in physically normal individuals who have not suffered illness or even injury. Some men ejaculate sperm into their bladder. These can be subsequently recovered from the urine, so microscopy of the urine has a place. Drugs may be helpful but generally couples with this problem will be treated by IVF. The urine can be carefully centrifuged and sperm-enriched fluid removed, washed and then used for IVF.

Human zona penetration and attachment tests To test the ability of a sperm to penetrate the zona ('shell') of the egg, it can be mixed with dead human eggs. This is largely experimental, available only in few research centres, and mostly of limited value. Another test involves counting the number of sperm attaching to the zona. Just before the sperm penetrate it, sperm stick to this outer shell and this can provide some information about sperm function and the chemical messages between sperm and egg.

Tests for DNA damage Some men produce sperm with extensive DNA damage and this can be seen under the microscope using special staining techniques. There are various tests, including the number of 'fragmented' sperm and various molecular tests. Many of these tests involve staining the sperm with fluorescent dyes. There is only a poor correlation between DNA damage and failure of fertilisation but it is associated with a poorer success rate during IVF.

Assessing reactive oxygen species (ROS) Around 25 per cent of infertile men have a raised ROS level. High levels seem to damage individual sperm cells, or immobilise them. Recently, scientists at the Cleveland Clinic in Chicago have shown that high ROS levels are associated with abnormal-looking sperm and postulate that ROS may damage spermatozoa. Freezing sperm may also result in raised levels of ROS, which is possibly why stored sperm are not as fertile. Tests for ROS levels require fairly complex laboratory equipment so they are not commonly done. It is suggested that vitamin treatments and possibly zinc dietary supplements may reduce ROS but the results are unclear.

Sperm proteomics There is rather insufficient research into sperm function, but one promising area is the investigation of the proteins (and genes) involved in sperm malfunction. Though currently limited, it holds promise for the future. We are slowly understanding what goes wrong during sperm development and how treatments might be improved. There are many processes involved in fertilisation. These include attraction of sperm to the egg, hypermotility (when the sperm approaches the egg), dispersion of the cells around the egg to allow access by sperm, attachment of sperm to the zona, egg penetration and the signals that initiate the development and fusion of the egg nucleus with sperm DNA.

Sperm-mucus interaction and the post-coital test (PCT) The post-coital test is an examination that has been discarded in many clinics but it has value. During a routine internal examination, approximately six to 36 hours after sex, a sample of cervical mucus is sucked into a small pipette. The presence of any still-moving sperm provides information about the ability of the sperm to survive inside the entrance to the uterus.

This test should be done in the first half of the menstrual cycle, just before ovulation, when the mucus should be watery and easily penetrated by sperm. It may help assessment of the man's fertility and whether his partner is ovulating and has a healthy cervix.

Because there are many reasons why a post-coital test may be negative this test is now less relevant. For example, women who have not ovulated may have rather thick, impenetrable mucus. But though many specialists have abandoned it, there is now evidence from researchers in Holland that a positive PCT is correlated with better chances of pregnancy in most couples.

Sperm-mucus interaction tests may also be done by taking a sample of mucus and putting it in contact with sperm under a microscope. If the sperm penetrate the mucus this suggests reasonable sperm function.

Hormone tests for men

Some men, particularly those whose testes are not producing sperm properly, may have abnormal hormone levels. The most important test is measurement of a man's follicle stimulating hormone (FSH). FSH is produced by the pituitary gland to stimulate the testes to make sperm. If the testes cannot produce sperm, the brain increases messages to the pituitary and more FSH is released. If the testes are unresponsive, FSH levels become high. Very high levels suggest that the testicle is not able to react to the pituitary's message, indicating that sperm manufacture, or spermatogenesis, may be failing or has stopped. High FSH levels often imply there will be no viable sperm.

It is useful to discover if the absence of sperm in the semen is due to a blockage in the tubes of the testis (in which case the FSH levels are unlikely to be raised) or whether the testis itself has failed. FSH may indicate that there is some sperm production, in which case it will help the specialist decide if one of the more complicated procedures associated with IVF is worthwhile. If a testis is still producing some sperm the recovery of some for microinjection (see ICSI, page 106) may be possible. Even with high FSH levels, men with testicular failure are still likely to produce male hormone (testosterone) so there are unlikely to be other problems with sexuality or virility.

Men may not produce sufficient FSH because the pituitary gland is damaged. In this rare event, administration of pituitary hormones (gonadotrophins) may be helpful.

Testicular biopsy

A small piece of tissue (biopsy) can be taken from one or both of the testes for examination. Usually this is done under general anaesthesia. Microscopy can determine whether the testes are producing some sperm normally and see if there are any viable sperm for advanced IVF procedures (see page 106). Sometimes the testicular tissue can be frozen for sperm storage.

Testicular biopsy is quite a big operation to recover bits of tissue; if repeated it can result in loss of testicular tissue. If excessive, this can reduce production of testosterone. Also it can cause some bleeding into the scrotum, so occasionally a stay in hospital overnight is necessary. Taking biopsies requires a scrotal incision, usually requiring stitches; it can be as uncomfortable as it sounds.

I once gave a public lecture to about 600 people about my research. Rather unwisely, I showed a photographic slide of a testicle being biopsied. There was a sudden movement in the middle of the second row of the packed lecture hall, and a man, rather prominently and quite noisily, fell off his chair onto the floor in a dead faint. This kind of thing can present a dilemma for a lecturer. I decided to move fairly rapidly to the next slide (a picture of a white rabbit eating lettuce). I then quickly clambered from the podium, over the first row of chairs to administer first aid. Then I continued my talk. Next day the *Daily Mail* reported that I showed more skill at primary care than infertility treatment.

Although testicular biopsy can be quite painful, tenderness can be relieved by wearing tight-fitting underwear or a jock strap to support the scrotum and testicles for a few days. Stitches are removed about a week later. It is best to avoid sexual activity for around two weeks.

Testicular mapping

This is a new approach for assessing testicular function, pioneered by Dr Turek in California. Many men with no sperm in the semen (azoospermia), may have some remaining in small areas of the testes where the tubules are most active. If these are identified, sperm can be surgically extracted to fertilise eggs using IVF. Mapping is done using local anaesthesia. A fine needle is inserted repeatedly into multiple sites in the testicle to build a 'map' of sperm-producing areas in either testis; this diagram can be used later to collect more sperm.

Testicular mapping is less damaging than a biopsy and less painful. Dr Turek claims remarkable pregnancy rates from the sperm of men previously considered completely sterile. He argues that mapping is better than repeated biopsy of the testis because, by not removing much testicular tissue, production of testosterone is not reduced. He says that although the testes don't exactly 'drop off' after biopsy, men clearly prefer not to impair their production of male hormone.

Thermography

This measures the temperature of the testes. Sometimes men with low sperm counts and prominent testicular veins (known as varicocoele) are thought have 'overheated' testes. Sperm production drops off when the testicles are at a higher than average temperature, which is why, it is thought, the testicles hang outside the body. Apparently this is irrelevant to elephants as they manage quite well with their testicles well inside the abdominal cavity. Anyway, whatever is thought of thermography (it understandably has never been tried in a large pachyderm, as far as I am aware) this test is of limited use.

Testicular ultrasound

An ultrasound examination of the testes is completely painless and may identify small cysts or, very occasionally, tumours which may be associated with damage to the testes.

Chromosome (karyotype) testing

Some men who are not producing enough normal sperm, or who are not producing any sperm, have a genetic abnormality. This may affect the male chromosome as some genes on the Y chromosome are missing or changed. Other chromosomal abnormalities include 'translocations', when parts of two different chromosomes stick together. This can be associated with infertility, usually because the sperm are incapable of fertilisation or because normal cell division of an embryo cannot take place. Translocations in either parent are also associated with miscarriage (see page 16).

Once the blood has been collected for chromosome analysis (karyotyping), it is cultured for two to four weeks. After staining individual white blood cells, an assessment of the chromosomes can be made. Karyotyping is valuable not only for various causes of male infertility, but some causes of unexplained infertility. Unfortunately, it cannot detect all genetic abnormalities associated with sperm production.

Tests for women

These include testing for ovulation, other hormone levels and chromosomal abnormalities, as well as investigations using different imaging techniques.

Ovulation

Tests to ensure you ovulate are the most important and often clinics use more than one for all their patients.

Progesterone The most widely tested hormone giving indirect evidence that you have ovulated. It is produced by the ovary during the second half of the cycle, after ovulation. Usually measured in 'nmols (nanomols) per litre', peak progesterone level is about 30nmols per litre (10 nanogms per litre) if ovulation occurs. It is at its highest about one week before the next menstrual period. The cells in the follicle that has just ovulated reduce oestrogen production and release progesterone, preparing the womb lining for an embryo, to provide a suitable environment for pregnancy.

Progesterone levels are not foolproof. Firstly, the test can be mistimed. The level of progesterone is highest about a week after ovulation for three to five days. It is therefore usual to take the test on day 21 of the cycle (roughly seven days before the next period starts). But if the cycle is irregular or if a period is a bit early or late, it is easy to miss the peak level. So it can help to repeat it several days after day 21 if a longer cycle is anticipated. The progesterone level falls sharply just before a period, so tests within a day or two of bleeding may be meaningless. Many couples become discouraged when they have a low reading, but it may simply mean that the first day of the period occurred sooner or later than expected.

Temperature charting This is no longer regarded as 'essential'. Temperature charts only provide limited information about ovulation.

Most women have a slight rise in body temperature shortly after ovulation (probably because the higher level of progesterone increases metabolism), but many normally ovulating women have no discernible change. So fertile women who study their temperature chart may be caused needless anxiety. Also, women who are not ovulating may notice a rise in temperature after the mid-cycle and wrongly conclude that ovulation is happening.

Some women hope charting their temperature will help them to time intercourse. The value of this is limited.

OVULATION DETECTION KITS

These kits can be obtained at pharmacies and measure levels of luteinising hormone (LH), the hormone produced by the pituitary which stimulates the ovary to ovulate. A slip of coated paper can be dipped in the first specimen of urine passed each morning; a colour change indicates increase in LH levels.

LH is secreted in larger amounts just before ovulation as the follicle matures in the ovary. When ovulation draws closer, the follicle containing an egg produces increased amounts of oestrogen. This enters the blood stream, circulates to the brain, 'telling' the pituitary that the ovary contains a mature follicle and is ready to release an egg. The resultant production of LH by the pituitary initiates ovulation.

These kits might seem like a good idea, but they are of limited value. They only test for the sudden surge of LH, which should occur about 36 hours before ovulation. Some women have an abnormal surge, but still ovulate. Others, particularly older women or those with polycystic ovaries, may produce high levels of LH but don't ovulate, confusing the test hopelessly. Sometimes the test just doesn't seem to work properly. Whatever the reason, these kits can increase the strain of infertility, because they encourage timed intercourse. Domination of one's sex life can make infertility more demanding and emotional. The kits are not cheap, at the time of writing they cost about £25 each.

Other hormone tests

Occasionally hormone levels may be measured during the early part of a menstrual cycle, thereby helping to pinpoint abnormalities affecting ovulation. Measurement of oestrogen, LH and FSH, and anti-mullerian hormone (AMH) are the most valuable.

On very rare occasions, low levels of FSH and LH may be found. These very occasionally indicate the need for hormone treatment. Much more usual are raised levels, commonly caused by polycystic ovaries. High levels of FSH indicate that the ovaries may be depleted of eggs and often predicts the onset of the menopause. Women with FSH raised much over 10 international units, and therefore likely to have some ovarian failure may not produce good eggs. Raised testosterone levels (which females also produce) may suggest that ovulation is not occurring – sometimes seen with polycystic ovary syndrome (PCOS).

The hormone prolactin, produced by the pituitary gland, may also be raised. Some women are worried that they have a high prolactin level, but if their periods are regular and if progesterone levels are consistent with ovulation, this is irrelevant. High prolactin levels may indicate PCOS. A very high level of prolactin suggests a rare tumour of the pituitary gland preventing ovulation.

Anti-mullerian hormone (AMH) This hormone has been known about since the 1940s, but is now used to predict fertility. At birth, a baby girl has one or two million tiny follicles in her ovaries, each containing an egg. Most follicles containing an immature egg disappear with age, so by puberty a girl has approximately 100,000–500,000 eggs left. Thereafter eggs are constantly lost whether or not she ovulates. By the age of 40, a woman may have around 10 per cent of her eggs left and the loss now continues more rapidly until the menopause. Follicles that are not lost develop to what is called the pre-antral stage. Cells lining these follicles produce AMH, so the level may indicate how many slowly maturing follicles remain; the theory is, the more follicles there are, the higher the AMH level. All of us age at different rates, so the loss of maturing follicles, and therefore eggs, varies in different women. AMH measurements give a clue to whether a woman is running out of eggs.

It all sounds too good to be true. One problem is that levels of AMH fluctuate, and there is considerable variation from person to person. Another is that measurements vary from lab to lab as the method for detecting this hormone is not standardised; even the way the blood is stored for the test can make a difference. Nevertheless AMH is a moderately good indicator of how many eggs are likely to be collected during IVF treatment, but it is not always such a good indicator of the chance of pregnancy. Although increasingly used, AMH measurement remains somewhat controversial because it does not necessarily predict the chances of a pregnancy. Even women with quite low levels occasionally get pregnant. There are other problems. As I mentioned earlier, high FSH levels are indicative of a lack of what is called 'ovarian reserve', or reduced follicles. But very often the levels of FSH and AMH do not correlate, for example, a woman can have high FSH levels but normal AMH levels.

AMH can be measured at any time during the cycle. It can predict, with some reliability, the ovarian reserve after a cancer treatment, or after surgery on the ovaries. It may predict the chances of hyperstimulation if gonadotrophins are used to stimulate the ovaries. AMH is often raised in people with PCOS. So it can help this diagnosis in some women; but may be less good at predicting ovarian reserve in those with PCOS.

AMH levels are usually measured in nanograms per litre but, confusingly, sometimes in picomols, giving a higher reading. A single measurement is usually inadequate to decide whether eggs are running out. You may wish to ask your doctor what levels are considered normal in the clinic you attend and how much variability may be expected.

Endometrial biopsy A small piece of the uterine lining (the endometrium) can be removed during the second half of the cycle and examined under the microscope. This helps to see if the lining is responding to the progesterone normally produced by the ovary after ovulation.

The best time for an endometrial biopsy is between days 18 and 28 day of a 28-day menstrual cycle. A small tube is gently inserted through the cervix and a tiny piece of uterine lining sucked away. It can cause brief, cramp-like period pain. Because some women are nervous, clinics may delay this procedure until laparoscopy under general anaesthesia (see page 42).

Endometrial biopsy is used increasingly to look for biochemical markers that may indicate whether the lining of the uterus is developing properly. These may show whether the uterus is capable of allowing an embryo to implant. Recently endometrial biopsy has gained a new significance as this tiny injury may itself help conception (see endometrial scratch, page 85).

Ovarian ultrasound High-frequency (inaudible) sound waves can be bounced off the ovaries and detected by an electronic transducer forming images that are displayed on a monitor.

The ovaries lie behind the bladder. As water is a good conductor of sound, pictures of an ovary can be obtained when the bladder is full and ultrasound is passed through the abdomen. So you may need to drink beforehand. Very accurate pictures of the ovaries can also be seen with a small transducer in the vagina, avoiding the discomfort of a full bladder and giving better photographs.

Ultrasound detects growing follicles and mature follicles ready to ovulate when they are approximately 2cm (½in) across. Repeated ultrasound may detect a sudden decrease in size suggesting an egg has been released. It is a key test for detecting polycystic ovaries, early pregnancy diagnosis, revealing cysts or ovarian damage due to endometriosis. Ultrasound can also assess fibroids in the uterus, but X-rays or magnetic resonance imaging (MRI) give more detailed pictures. In recent years ultrasound has been used to assess whether the Fallopian tubes are open, using a special solution – the so-called HyCoSy test. This test is not reliable in my experience and X-rays or laparoscopy are more accurate.

Testing the Fallopian tubes and the uterus
This can be carried out using a number of techniques.

Hysterosalpingogram (HSG) This is an X-ray of the uterus and Fallopian tubes. It is unduly neglected because some doctors think it has been superseded. But it provides information difficult to get in other ways, moreover, it is easy to do and inexpensive.

The X-ray is done at a vaginal examination. The doctor inserts a thin tube through the cervix. The instrument that fits inside the cervix is no larger than a ballpoint pen refill. A small amount of dye is injected into the uterus, and its progress through the uterus and Fallopian tubes is monitored on a television screen; about six X-ray photos may be taken. X-rays reveal whether the tubes are open and the shadows they provide can also give excellent views of the inside of the uterus, and the lining of the tubes. With modern X-ray equipment and carefully taken images, it is possible to detect scarring in the wall of the tubes; the detail obtained provides invaluable information.

Some clinics organise an HSG as soon as possible after your first clinic visit. When you return for your follow-up appointment there will be a detailed assessment of the tubes and uterus.

With digital-enhancing equipment a computer image makes the procedure simpler and more informative. HSG used to have a reputation for being painful, but this is now largely untrue. Many women do not even realise that the test has started or finished. Sometimes the insertion of the tube can cause a little discomfort, but no worse than a period pain. Persistent pain hours after the HSG can indicate infection and any woman who experiences this should contact the hospital no matter how late at night it might be.

HSG is excellent at identifying adhesions inside the uterus, fibroids, scarring of the uterine muscle and polyps. It can also outline congenital abnormalities, which are not uncommon causes of infertility. In the area where the tubes join the uterus the internal plumbing is extremely delicate and small. HSG is far more effective than laparoscopy (see page 42) in revealing any scar tissue or polyps in the tubes. A good X-ray also reveals changes in the tubal lining and its folds. This is important because so often there is tubal disease even though the tubes are not blocked. This knowledge helps inform decisions about treatment. Such scarring can make an ectopic pregnancy (implanting in one or other Fallopian tube) more likely.

I have seen so many women who have undergone IVF unsuccessfully. Frequently they have been told they have 'unexplained infertility'. All too often an HSG has not been done, or done inadequately. When HSG is performed properly, we often uncover a clear reason for the failure of earlier IVF attempts. As most of these contributing factors are entirely correctable, it is a great pity that more emphasis is not placed on getting good quality HSG X-rays before IVF treatment.

Magnetic resonance imaging (MRI) An accurate but rather expensive way of occasionally assessing the pelvic organs. The part of the body to be examined is placed in an intense magnetic field, produced by a large coil in a cylinder that totally surrounds the body. It is a painless procedure, but it can be slightly unnerving as the machine makes a considerable noise. With the latest equipment, MRI gives high-quality images, far better than those achieved using ultrasound. They are not as good as a high-quality X-ray, but MRI does not involve any exposure to X-radiation.

MRI produces detailed images of your insides, and is probably not used often enough. In particular, it gives evidence of damage to the wall of the uterus and scar tissue in the muscle. We sometimes use it when we suspect we are dealing with the condition called adenomyosis (see page 133), or sometimes to investigate cysts. Adenomyosis is a frequent cause of infertility and may cause painful periods. It is quite common in older women.

Because MRI is relatively expensive it is mainly used only when there is suspicion that the uterine wall is abnormal. Patients who have slightly irregular, but chronically painful periods and women who bleed during the menstrual cycle, are rather more likely to have adenomyosis.

Laparoscopic examination Laparoscopy is the single most important test for female infertility. In my view it nearly always should be considered before entering an IVF programme, unless it is definitely known that a woman has no Fallopian tubes, or that there is no possibility of corrective surgery. Sadly, the bodies that run the NHS do not agree with my view and the NICE guidelines (see page 20) have tried to limit the number of laparoscopies done to save NHS money. Laparoscopy is done under general anaesthesia, normally as a day case. A thin telescope is inserted into the abdominal cavity through a small hole made in the navel. Carbon dioxide, passed into the abdomen, separates the organs so that they can be seen easily. The telescope is no thicker than a fountain pen, but with the improvement in modern optics superb photographs can be taken. A surgeon can use the laparoscope to inspect the outside of the uterus, and to see if the tubes are open by injecting coloured dye. The whole procedure may take anything from 15–45 minutes, and rather longer if it is being used for keyhole surgery (for example to release the Fallopian tubes from adhesions). An endometrial biopsy can be taken at the same time.

You will normally find two or three small dressings on the abdomen afterwards. One covers a single stitch in the navel, the other a tiny hole near the pubic hairline. This second hole is used to place any fine probes shaped like small knitting needles into the abdominal cavity to move tissues around to get a better view. Laparoscopy usually causes very little pain or discomfort, although some women may feel unwell and need to rest in bed for 24 hours.

The benefits of a laparoscopy

- It is the best way to determine whether the tubes have been damaged.
- It uniquely shows adhesions in the pelvis that may prevent pregnancy.
- It gives a direct view of the ovaries and, if done in the second half of the woman's cycle, enables the surgeon to see whether there has been recent ovulation.
- It gives a good idea of the size of the ovaries. This is important because women with very small ovaries are more likely to produce few eggs during stimulation for IVF.
- It is the best and usually the only way to detect endometriosis.
- It gives an excellent view of the outside of the uterus and may help to detect fibroids or a congenital problem in the womb.
- It can detect relevant scarring elsewhere in the abdomen, in particular, adhesions around the liver, which can indicate previous infection that has caused normally undetectable damage to the tubes.
- It facilitates the taking of small pieces of tissue (biopsies) or fluids that give useful pathological or bacteriological information.
- It allows the surgeon to introduce small scissors, a diathermy needle or a laser, which can be used to treat a range of conditions from adhesions to polycystic ovaries.

After laparoscopy more women immediately conceive than would be expected by chance. Historically, up to about 15 per cent of our patients with open tubes conceive within three months of laparoscopy.

Hysteroscopy A small telescope, called a hysteroscope, can be passed into the uterus through the vagina. It is a good way to detect polyps, fibroids, adhesions or congenital abnormalities that may

COMMON SIDE EFFECTS OF LAPAROSCOPY

- **Soreness in the abdomen**
- **Soreness in one or other shoulder** This is because the carbon dioxide injected into the abdomen can irritate the nerves to the abdominal lining, which also supply the shoulder area.
- **Vaginal bleeding** This may occur if the surgeon manipulates the cervix during injection of the dye to check the tubes. It may last two or three days and sometimes longer.

be suspected following the results of an HSG. It can also be used to treat some of these conditions. This usually needs a quick general anaesthetic on a day visit to the hospital. It does not replace the HSG as this gives detailed information of a different kind.

Tuboscopy and falloscopy A fine telescope can be inserted through the abdominal wall under general anaesthetic to inspect the inside of the Fallopian tube. Tuboscopy can be combined with laparoscopy. It is of limited value, except possibly to the surgeon who may charge large fees for it. An alternative is a falloscopy, namely the passage of a very fine telescope into the Fallopian tube via the vagina and uterus. I do not know the going rate for falloscopy. It probably has even less value than tuboscopy and is included here for completeness[1]. These tests may be slightly helpful in assessing the lining of the tubes following ectopic pregnancy.

Chromosome (karyotype) testing

Like men, women may also have chromosomal abnormalities causing infertility. These women may not ovulate or have, for example, repeated miscarriages. If a chromosomal abnormality is suspected, this can be detected using blood tests (see page 35). Until recently chromosome abnormalities were totally untreatable. However, some

---

1   I remember one surgeon being asked by his anaesthetist what he expected to see by doing a falloscopy. He replied, 'Fifty pound notes'.

infertile women (particularly those who miscarry frequently) have a chromosomal abnormality that may be passed to some of their embryos. Preimplantation genetic screening, or PGS (see page 94), can sometimes be used to choose a normal embryo to avoid miscarriage.

Dilation and curettage

Occasionally women who have difficulty conceiving are brought into hospital for a 'womb scrape'. Dilation and curettage, or D&C, probably does no harm, but is generally useless unless an endometrial biopsy is carried out to give information about the uterine lining. It is often done in the vain belief that it makes it easier to conceive.

Trace elements, vitamins, hair testing

Some clinics prey on the fears of women by offering blood tests, or tests on hair or tissue, to detect dietary and other deficiencies. I cannot emphasis enough how strongly I feel about these tests, which may be a confidence trick. Typically, I have heard of women having locks of hair examined for trace elements for which they are charged quite large sums of money. The results, which are difficult to validate, may be said to show an absence of zinc, magnesium, cadmium, vitamins or some other substances that in most cases have little proved value in treating human fertility.

Chapter 4: In vitro fertilisation

IVF is the process by which egg and sperm are mixed in a plastic dish outside the body. Within 2–5 days of fertilisation, the embryo is placed in the uterus (before five days of development, no organs have formed and the embryo is invisible to the naked eye). Treatment involves removing eggs from the ovaries and the collection of sperm from a partner.

IVF should only be considered after serious attempts at making a diagnosis to understand the cause of the infertility has been made. Depending on diagnosis, it must be remembered that there are treatments that are more successful than IVF and less expensive. Where indicated these should be tried first. Sometimes, after exhaustive investigation, no cause for infertility may be found and this is regarded as an indication for IVF. However, good research does not show better chances of pregnancy compared with simpler management for most cases of unexplained infertility (see page 20).

Unfortunately, IVF is frequently seen as a panacea for infertility. Far too many couples attempt it when other straightforward, cheaper treatments are more applicable. When a cause for the infertility is not found IVF may be useful because it may help understand the underlying cause of infertility.

IVF is not a first option

Due to massive publicity, IVF has false reputation as the only answer to infertility. However, it is the most demanding of all procedures in reproductive medicine and actually less likely to result in a live birth than many alternatives. Also, strictly speaking, IVF is not even a 'treatment' for infertility as it does not alter the underlying cause; it is simply a one-off attempt to help someone to have a baby. While IVF can be repeated, the cause of infertility is usually unchanged. IVF has, however, revolutionised the treatment of very many infertile people who have no serious alternative. It also has improved our knowledge about many causes of infertility, so is useful diagnostically if the cause is obscure.

IVF is occasionally confused with artificial insemination (AI), which usually involves placing sperm directly into a woman's vagina or uterus with a syringe (see page 122). Some women avoid a doctor and self-inseminate. Of course, a key problem is how they obtain sperm from an untested donor who is free of infection[1].

I believe IVF is not a first option. My contention is over half of those referred to IVF clinics may be treated by alternatives. Too frequently no systematic assessment of the medical condition of the patient is made. Referring GPs sometimes need to educate themselves about fertility treatments (usually ignored in most medical student teaching programmes). A good GP will have the information and sensitivity to make sound judgments about whether his or her patient would most benefit from IVF treatment, rather than from an alternative. Sometimes, of course, patients themselves push for IVF when there may be a more suitable treatment.

Even specialists in reproductive medicine tend to offer IVF before it is proven to be necessary. Too many couples start on an IVF programme before complete medical investigation. This is doubly unfortunate. First, IVF can fail because there is an underlying condition (for example, a uterine abnormality) that needs treatment and may prevent pregnancy even if an embryo is transferred to the womb. Secondly, robust treatment of the actual cause is avoided, when this may mean better chances of conception. I cannot overstate the importance of diagnosing the true cause of infertility if at all possible. The investigations that should be done before IVF are discussed in Chapter 3.

---

1   Much has been made of the 'terrible risks' unmarried women may take by finding a willing friend to donate semen. Given some knowledge of human behaviour these risks may be exaggerated. Needless to say, artificial insemination simply requires sperm to be placed in the vagina or uterus. But clinics are seemingly making huge profits even out of this simple procedure. A single friend of mine has just be quoted £11,000 for a course of three cycles of artificial insemination. It is not surprising then that a 'willing friend' might suddenly seem rather attractive.

When should you consider IVF?

First, and most important, both partners should have a continuing discussion about whether you really want to undergo what can be a demanding and fraught treatment. It may surprise readers, but I have regrettably seen many situations where, at the last minute, one partner, having agreed to undergo IVF and signed informed consent earlier, has refused consent to egg collection at the last minute. On occasion, when all is ready after successful embryo culture, another refused to have the embryos transferred. In addition, I have encountered at least six patients who sadly suddenly requested an abortion after an IVF pregnancy had been successfully established.

Medical reasons for IVF

In strict medical terms, IVF is clearly appropriate in the following situations.

- When the Fallopian tubes are so badly damaged that tubal surgery has failed or is not worth contemplating, IVF is the only satisfactory treatment. However, it is often not necessary if there is relatively minor disease of the Fallopian tubes. Then it may be worth asking your GP to seek an expert opinion as to whether tubal surgery by a suitably experienced surgeon might be justified.
- If a man has an abnormal or low sperm count, but the sperm are still potentially capable of fertilising an egg, IVF is undoubtedly the ideal course of action as manipulation of the sperm in the laboratory can increase the chance of fertilisation.
- If a women is not ovulating and attempts to use drugs to stimulate ovulation adequately have repeatedly failed. IVF may be indicated in polycystic ovary disease, for example. However, IVF is less suitable for women who produce very few eggs or those of very poor quality, usually only after very heavy stimulation (see page 54). Then IVF with a donor egg from another woman may be the best alternative (see page 101).
- For women with endometriosis, although stimulation of the ovaries in these patients will increase the circulating hormone level of oestrogen,

which in turn may stimulate the endometriosis and can make it more severe. It is not uncommon for women with endometriosis to find that symptoms of pain and irregular bleeding increase after unsuccessful IVF treatment. Endometriosis may be treated surgically and by hormone treatments, which may be more successful.

- In cases of unexplained infertility, where proper attempts to diagnose infertility have been unsuccessful and the cause remains unexplained, IVF can be valuable. In general, IVF may help to establish the cause of failure to conceive. In older women, where 'unexplained infertility' may be because the ovaries are incapable of producing normal eggs, IVF has a low success rate.

- When there is a problem in the cervix or severe scarring of the top of the vagina, IVF may be indicated. Once an embryo is obtained it can be placed directly into the uterine cavity.

- Most importantly, when there are multiple factors causing infertility, usually affecting both the man and the woman, IVF is generally the most effective treatment. So, for example, if there is a minor sperm problem combined with a minor problem of scarring of the Fallopian tubes, IVF greatly increases the chances of fertilisation and pregnancy.

- For couples carrying single defects who are also at high risk of having genetically abnormal babies. Typically this may include diseases such as cystic fibrosis or muscular dystrophy. Using preimplantation genetic screening (see PGS, page 94), an assessment of whether or not a particular embryo is free of the genetic defect carried in that family can be made, and a healthy embryo can be selected and placed in the uterus. This treatment is sometimes used for patients with chromosomal abnormalities that cause miscarriages.

When is IVF likely to be useless?
There are some couples for whom IVF is likely to be of little help.

- When a man is not producing any sperm. If the testes are not producing any of the cells that make mature spermatozoa, there is no chance of IVF working. One alternative is the use of donor semen (see page 115).

- When the uterus has been removed by hysterectomy there is no prospect of bearing a child. For these women, the only possibility is adoption or surrogacy (see page 105). Uterine transplantation from a healthy woman has been done in Sweden and the UK, but it is a complex operation and not without risk. It may be possible to take an egg from the ovaries (if these are still intact), fertilise it outside the body and produce a surrogate pregnancy in another woman.
- Some rare infections of the uterus such as tuberculosis make implantation and subsequent pregnancy impossible.
- Where severe adhesions inside the uterine cavity largely obliterate it (Asherman's syndrome). In its most severe, untreatable form, embryo transfer will fail and therefore IVF is generally not worth trying. Other rare conditions of the uterus include congenital absence of the womb, or serious deformity of the cavity.
- When the ovaries are very scarred, extensively cystic or not capable of producing an egg because of scar tissue.
- When the ovaries are failing to produce any eggs, or when women are in the older age group and post-menopausal. The only possibility is an egg from a donor (see page 101).
- In women with severe bowel adhesions around the ovaries as this makes any form of egg collection a life-threatening procedure.

The cost of IVF

I regret deeply the commercial market surrounding IVF. In the UK, the NHS is much to blame for two reasons. Firstly, it has ignored how serious is the pain of infertility affecting so many couples, and that this symptom indicates underlying disease processes which are fully worthy of treatment in any democratic society with proper access to health care. So often, it does not take the needs of people who are infertile seriously. They are shunted into the private sector where IVF has become dominated by a highly profitable industry. Unquestionably, IVF should not cost nearly as much as what is commonly charged – the combination of the desperation of patients, combined with the avarice of some practitioners is deeply corrosive. This changes attitudes at every level. Of course, there are very scrupulous, honest, kind and ethical doctors in this field operating in excellent clinics, but a kind of cartel often exists. Each clinic recognises what another may charge, and as there are so many people who wish to have treatment, there is little incentive to charge much less than another centre. Eventually we see the consequences – clinics advertising on the London Underground with dubious ethicality for example, or exaggerated claims promoted in the media about procedures which 'Offer new hope for childless couples', patients paying for procedures that are effectively research projects with no proven value, or claims being made for some new treatment, which has been marketed well before any serious randomised controlled trials have been published or evaluated.

Secondly, the NHS is much to blame because it, too, operates a market. NHS centres do not charge what the treatment actually costs to deliver, but rather what it hopes the market will bear. The NHS is cash-strapped so any profit is much sought after. By NHS clinics charging NHS purchasing authorities large fees, the number of treatment cycles that the purchasers with a fixed budget can afford to buy has to be reduced – thus limiting many patients to just one cycle of treatment with consequently an overall lower chance of success. Thereafter patients failing treatment are forced into the private sector, often into private clinics ironically operated by the same practitioners who treated them initially under the NHS. Here is real potential for a conflict of interests.

Regrettably, the regulatory authority, the HFEA has done far too little to change what is charged both in the private sector, and also in the NHS. But it is ludicrous that an NHS cycle of treatment may cost £1,000 in some parts of the country and the same treatment in others over £5,000. (For further discussion of the costs of IVF see pages 143–144.)

Chapter 5: How is IVF done?

I apologise this seems a dry description of the IVF process but it may help some readers, new to the procedures involved, to understand each step.

Before treatment, and following routine fertility investigations, several specific tests should be carried out.

Hormone levels should be rechecked particularly the level of the follicle stimulating hormone (FSH). If the FSH is much above 10 international units, then attempts to stimulate the ovaries may be a complete failure. Measurement of anti-mullerian hormone (AMH) is now almost routine; a low result may also indicate the possibility of an inadequate response to ovarian stimulation. The uterine cavity should be examined if this has not been done recently. A probe such as a fine plastic tube should be passed through the cervix to make sure that an embryo transfer will not be difficult. Your doctor should also check the hysterosalpingogram (HSG) X-rays personally rather than merely reading a radiological report. I say this because some radiological units may not make a detailed assessment of the HSG. You may also be given drugs such as clomiphene in a prior menstrual cycle which may indicate that your ovaries are capable of responding to the drugs used during IVF treatment. Sperm counts should be rechecked and sperm function tests should be run and the motility of the sperm assessed.

The stages of IVF

Several eggs are usually required to increase the likelihood of a viable embryo. Most IVF treatment involves giving injections of the hormone FSH to encourage the ovaries to produce more than the one egg. In exceptional cases up to 40 eggs can be obtained in one cycle, but it is very rare for all of them to fertilise and develop into normal embryos. Having a large number of eggs is not usually advantageous as overstimulation increases the chance of producing abnormal eggs. In an average, successful treatment, around 10–15 eggs are most frequently produced but older women, or those with reduced ovarian function, tend to respond less. Different IVF clinics will have varying approaches so my description below will vary. There is no ideal method of stimulation and most clinics give a regime which seems most successful in their hands. The preparations of FSH most widely used in the UK are called Gonal-F and Puregon. Menogon, Menopur and Merional also contain luteinising hormone (LH) and some clinics give these drugs because they may give a more 'natural' response in some women who are difficult to treat. It is reasonable to ask your doctors why they think the stimulation they offer you is the most suitable.

Suppression of ovarian function

One way of increasing the chance of satisfactory ovarian stimulation is to induce a brief, temporary 'menopause' for two or three weeks. Drugs such as Nafarelin, Buserelin or Goserelin – so-called pituitary agonists – are commonly used. They prevent the pituitary gland from producing FSH. Consequently the ovaries not only stop ovulating, but also stop growing follicles in which eggs develop. This seems surprising, but this usually makes the ovary more sensitive to FSH given by injections.

In the UK one drug commonly used to suppress ovarian function is Suprefact (Buserelin). This is normally sniffed every four to six hours throughout the day, usually one sniff into each nostril, which allows the drug to be very rapidly absorbed. Women who cannot sniff – perhaps because of a cold – or those who have very poor nasal absorption of the drug, can be given injections.

Cetrotide and Orgalutran, also given by injection, are alternatives. They are called pituitary antagonists; they block release of FSH and LH from the pituitary gland. Their effect can be gained by a single depot injection. This approach is more popular in the USA and some parts of Europe.

Curiously, although all these drugs work by suppressing pituitary function, in the first few days after their administration they frequently stimulate it, so that the pituitary briefly produces more FSH than normal (the 'flare' effect). Some clinics use this effect and injections of FSH are then given before the pituitary is suppressed, cutting down the amount needed. This particular 'short protocol' approach may be useful if you do not respond well to injections of FSH. It has gained acceptance for women in their late thirties or early forties.

Drugs which suppress the ovaries are frequently started the day after menstruation begins. However, some units prefer starting in the second half of the cycle, roughly one week before the period is due.

Drugs acting on the pituitary can cause headaches; a few people get quite severe hot flushes, vaginal dryness and mood changes. Rarely, slight vaginal bleeding can occur. These symptoms are unpleasant and uncomfortable, but are not dangerous, disappearing when the drugs are stopped. On rare occasions, suppression of the pituitary function continues for a few weeks after stopping drugs. Some women have an irregular cycle or two if they do not conceive.

Ovarian stimulation

The ovaries are usually suppressed within two weeks of these treatments. Confirmation that the ovaries are not 'active' is made by ultrasound examinations, which shows no developing follicles. Blood tests may confirm the ovaries are producing little oestrogen, further evidence that they are quiescent. Once the ovaries are suppressed injections of FSH are given. The recombinant FSH drugs Gonal-F or Puregon are now mostly used. These are given by daily injection and have virtually totally replaced the older drugs Pergonal and Metrodin[1].

---

1 Pergonal frequently contained unwanted proteins, occasionally causing adverse reactions. It is said that these drugs were originally obtained by extracting the active hormones from the urine of menopausal women – who usually have high levels of FSH and sometimes LH in their system. Apparently the most convenient source for the many gallons of menopausal urine needed were Italian nunneries. This account was hotly denied by the drug company, possibly because the industry saw the irony of the Catholic Church aiding a therapy to which it is not exactly favourably disposed.

The modern, genetically engineered (recombinant) drugs appear to be safer because they do not contain proteins that might cause allergies (see footnote, page 54) but they are more expensive. Older women, who generally do not respond so well to ovarian stimulation, may need more of these drugs.

Assessing follicle development

Egg collection is carried out just before ovulation is expected. If eggs are collected earlier, they may not fertilise. Before ovulation, the follicles containing the egg gradually become responsive to LH. But in women whose pituitary has been suppressed for example, with Buserelin (see page 53), no LH is produced. So drugs are needed to mature the eggs sufficiently for fertilisation; human chorionic gonadotrophin (hCG), a compound similar in structure to LH, is injected approximately 36 hours before the egg collection; hCG is as effective and cheaper than LH.

If given too early, the egg may not mature properly; if it is given too late, ovulation may result in eggs being lost completely. Some clinics do regular hormone tests to measure oestrogen levels during stimulation, as this indicates how well the follicles are responding to the FSH, and to time the hCG injection. Ultrasound is usually done repeatedly to assess the growth of follicles. When the biggest follicle is about 17–20mm across, ovulation is imminent, and it is time for the hCG injection, usually 10–14 days after starting FSH.

A few clinics are increasingly reverting to so-called 'natural cycle' IVF, which is how some of us used to do it 35 years ago (see page 80). At that time IVF seemed more effective when we stimulated the ovaries to obtain a substantial number of eggs in one 'go'. However, it was recognised that heavy stimulation of the ovaries might produce eggs that were not properly matured. Research done by the Genesis Research Trust showed that animal or human ovaries stimulated with large amounts of gonadotrophins (FSH) produced more genetically abnormal eggs. This, incidentally, shows the value of animal research. In mice, the number of chromosomal abnormalities in eggs after FSH treatment was proportional to the dose given; the more FSH, the more the eggs were abnormal.

Some women just do not respond well to FSH. So clinics may give no stimulus to the ovaries (perhaps beyond a dose of clomiphene by mouth) other than a single injection of hCG to trigger ovulation (see page 120).

Egg collection

Eggs are usually collected using vaginal ultrasound. The ultrasound probe gives an image of each ovary. A needle is then placed through the top of the vagina and guided into each follicle. Eggs are sucked into a small test tube, and then handed to the embryologist. This usually requires just light general or local anaesthesia.

It is not always possible to get all the eggs – or sometimes even a single egg. But about 97 per cent of attempts at egg collection yield at least one egg, unless there is severe ovarian disease. It is not uncommon to give an antibiotic for a few days after egg collection to prevent infection. Recovery is usually swift; most women leave the clinic within 2–4 hours of collection. Serious pain or soreness is rare, but as you may feel a bit light-headed, it is best to be accompanied from the clinic.

Exceptionally eggs may be collected by laparoscopy if, for example, the ovaries cannot easily be seen by vaginal or abdominal ultrasound. This requires a telescope to be inserted into the abdomen under a general anaesthetic.

Egg culture, sperm preparation and fertilisation

Once the eggs have been collected how they are kept is critical. They are carefully placed in a special fluid and examined under a microscope in the operating room where they have just been obtained. Once assessed, they are placed in a culture containing precisely measured amounts of the chemicals (proteins, hormones, energy-releasing materials). The eggs are then put into an incubator in closely controlled conditions resembling those in the body.

Culture media vary from unit to unit but all have the basic constituents required for fertilisation and early growth. Maternal serum may be added, because this provides a balance of some essential ingredients.

Meanwhile, shortly before the eggs are collected, the male partner will produce semen. Clinics keep a room available for this purpose. Men often find masturbation during IVF difficult and the emotional pressure can often cause failure to ejaculate. If this is likely to be a difficulty, it is possible to arrange to freeze and store semen before treatment (see page 111), but thawed semen may not always be as fertile.

Sperm are washed and all debris commonly present in semen removed. The fluid is diluted and sperm counted under a microscope. About 4–8 hours after egg collection, they will be mixed with the eggs and returned to the incubator. Often there are unanticipated problems with the sperm, perhaps too few or too weakly motile. IVF usually requires several thousand well-functioning sperm to guarantee fertilisation of just one egg. That may seem a large number, but even healthy men may have surprisingly inefficient testicles, possibly why a normal ejaculate contains several million sperm to maintain the human race. On the occasions when there are less than a few thousand, or sperm are not normal, help may be needed. This normally involves the microinjection of sperm into the egg (see ICSI, page 106).

Assessment of fertilisation

Cultured eggs are often inspected microscopically about 18 hours after they have been mixed with the sperm. This may be the only time at which it is possible to observe definite signs of fertilisation. What the embryologist will be looking for are two pronuclei – the nucleus of the egg and of the fertilising sperm – but they are only visible at this stage. It seems amazing, but if left later it is quite common for some unfertilised eggs to divide into several cells, a process known as 'parthenogenetic cleavage'. Such embryos are not capable of producing a human birth as far as we know, but researchers have achieved 'virgin birth' in mice. In the past, unless cultured eggs were carefully observed, unfertilised, parthenogenetically cleaved eggs might be transferred to the uterus giving all kinds of false hopes. If more than one sperm penetrates the egg (so-called 'polyspermic' fertilisation) an embryo that will not survive is formed. Polyspermy is more common when the eggs are abnormal because the usual safety mechanism fails.

Embryo assessment

The embryos usually divide into at least 2–4 cells by 48 hours. At some time from then on they will normally be ready for transfer to the uterus. An embryologist will check again to ensure that they look normal. If there are doubts about their development a further check is made 24 hours later. This may not affect the chances of successful pregnancy. If an embryo seems seriously abnormal, it may be discarded rather than risk an event like a miscarriage. Many clinics nowadays culture some embryos for longer than two or three days. Transferring embryos at five days, when they should have developed into a blastocyst, gives a higher chance of pregnancy. This may seem a considerable advantage, but many embryos do not develop in culture and become blastocysts, so the chance of having an embryo to transfer is reduced.

The so-called Embryoscope is a recent innovation (see page 92), which photographs the progress of embryonic development. Claims are made that this enables embryologists to choose the best embryos. The excitement that greeted this patented device typifies the exaggerated claims with which every innovation in IVF seems to be accompanied; commercial interests certainly played their part. Possibly the biggest advantage of this device is that it prevents embryos being exposed to environmental fluctuations every time a culture oven is opened.

All clinics assess embryo quality by looking at embryos down a conventional, low-power microscope, an imperfect way of predicting whether an embryo is capable of further development. A normal embryo tends to have divided into cells of equal size that are round and smooth, but this is no guarantee of normality. In general, symmetrically cleaved embryos are more likely to become babies. Some embryos may have abnormal numbers of cells or be unequal in size. This may be just because the embryo is dividing at the time of inspection or because the cells are breaking up. Some embryos are very fragmented, with many little pieces of unequal size and shape. However, even very abnormal-looking embryos can occasionally produce a pregnancy. Surprisingly, an abnormal-looking embryo, if transferred to the womb, does not seem to give an increased risk of an abnormal infant.

Many clinical embryologists reassure patients that their embryos are 'excellent'. Many even give a grading of one to four with further subgrades. It is reasonable to grade embryos for scientific purposes or to use this for quality control, but it is wrong to place serious emphasis on grading when speaking to patients. Even most normal-looking embryos are frequently not capable of becoming a baby. Telling somebody that they have 'excellent embryos' following a crude observation – gives no indication of what is happening at the molecular level where any abnormalities mostly exist. It is rather like looking at a man's face on the Piccadilly Line on the London Underground and surmising that he looks intelligent, brutal, dishonest or stupid. No embryologist can truly assess the quality of any microscopic human embryo by gazing fondly at it.

Embryos which divide faster may sometimes be slightly more likely to become a baby. If an embryo has divided into only two to four cells three days after fertilisation, then success is less likely than if an embryo has divided into eight or ten cells. However, this is only a rule of thumb and even slowly dividing embryos can become healthy babies.

Embryo transfer

Pregnancy is more likely when more than one embryo is placed in the uterus simultaneously because many normally fertilised human embryos do not develop into babies. To overcome this natural loss it has been standard practice to transfer several embryos (if available) into the uterus simultaneously. But the transfer of more than one embryo risks twins, or occasionally triplets. Multiple pregnancy carries high risks of the death of a baby, serious abnormality or a very premature baby. Multiple embryo transfer is tempting but should be avoided and HFEA regulations stipulate that wherever possible only single embryos should be transferred. Exceptions are made for older women or those who have already failed IVF because their embryos are likely to be less viable.

There are no absolute restrictions on transfer in most countries. It seems amazing that in some parts of the USA, four, five or even six embryos are occasionally transferred – success at all odds. Market forces push medical practice into dangerous ethical areas.

When an embryo has grown sufficiently, it is put into a fine plastic tube with a droplet of culture fluid. After a brief vaginal examination, the tube is inserted through the cervix, and the fluid is injected with extreme care into the uterus. Nearly all clinics conduct embryo transfer with you lying on your back. This is straightforward and hardly felt. Once the transfer has taken place, it is usual to suggest you remain lying down for 10–30 minutes. This may help the embryo to 'stay put', but there is no good evidence for this. Indeed research suggests that no amount of normal movement will dislodge the embryo.

Some units have adopted the practice used at Hammersmith Hospital, which ensures that the embryo catheter is in the right place inside the uterine cavity. Abdominal ultrasound is used whilst the catheter is being inserted and the tip of the catheter can be seen on the screen with its blob of fluid containing an embryo. Once this is done, the catheter is checked under a microscope by the embryologist to confirm that the embryo has left the catheter. If an embryo is still in the tubing, it is easy to repeat the procedure.

Days after embryo transfer women frequently worry about moving around too much. Many are so frightened of losing their embryos that they talk about lying rigidly in bed – one lawyer described to me how she 'lay at attention like a private in the Marines'. That seems totally unnecessary. An embryo implants several days after it has been transferred and there is no evidence at all that routine activities have any effect. Think about it – nobody would ever get pregnant if average movement compromised conception. My advice is 'don't regard yourself as an invalid'. Possibly take things easy for a few days for your own peace of mind, perhaps staying away from work for a day or two and avoiding sex for two weeks. It may be best not to travel overseas so you can stay in touch with the clinic if you suddenly feel worried.

Progesterone support

Developing pregnancies require the uterine lining (endometrium) to be fit for implantation, and after ovulation the ovary produces progesterone to grow it properly. If your pituitary gland has been suppressed with drugs, the ovaries may not produce enough progesterone, so this is usually given after embryo transfer. Many clinics administer an initial dose of progesterone by injection for a few days and later in a vaginal pessary. This may be continued for about two weeks. It is controversial whether continuing longer helps; it may suppress the onset of a period and a woman may think she is pregnant simply because her uterine lining cannot bleed.

In a woman whose pituitary gland is not suppressed there is less reason to give progesterone as an ovary is capable of producing large amounts of progesterone, particularly if there were several follicles before egg collection. Most units still give an injection of hCG (which is possibly unnecessary) but this stimulates your punctured follicles to produce progesterone.

Pregnancy testing

Even after all this and a successful transfer the odds are against getting pregnant. Many embryos, perhaps nearly 80 per cent, are lost before the menstrual period is due. They may have looked normal under a microscope, but it is likely that they were poorly developed in some way and incapable of producing a pregnancy. This happens in fertile people too, as many embryos produced naturally are also incapable of subsequent development.

Some clinics do not test for pregnancy at all; others ask you to send in a urine sample. Some take blood on day 12 or 14 after transfer – the earliest a pregnancy is usually detectable. Sometimes the hormone levels may indicate pregnancy, but are rather lower than normal. This suggests a pregnancy which may not be implanting completely. If, after further testing, these hormones remain low, it is probable that the pregnancy is only 'biochemical', meaning it is likely to miscarry at an early stage. Occasionally, a low test result can mean that the pregnancy has implanted in a Fallopian tube and is ectopic (see page 64). This requires further blood tests and ultrasound examinations. Conversely, a high level of pregnancy hormone (human chorionic gonadotrophin/hCG) suggests the possibility of twins.

Chapter 6: The risks of IVF

As with any medical procedure, IVF does carry some risks. These include abnormalities and multiple births, certain long-term risks, ectopic pregnancy, ovarian hyperstimulation (OHSS) and irregular periods. IVF has been linked to an increased chance of developing some cancers and the research is discussed here. Finally, the emotional challenge involved with IVF can be considerable.

Abnormal babies and multiple births

At the time of writing about 5,500,000 babies have been born around the world after IVF. There is no definite evidence that they are more at risk from abnormalities than naturally conceived babies. Indeed, after IVF certain abnormalities (including chromosome problems, like Down's syndrome, for example) are less common. IVF babies may have more problems at birth, and stillbirths may be more common. This may not be due to IVF itself but because women who conceive through IVF are more likely to have a 'high risk' pregnancy.

Transfer of more than one embryo risks multiple pregnancy and twins are more likely to have birth defects. The US Center for Disease Control (CDC) published the results of IVF in 147,000 IVF procedures in the USA in 2010[1]. There were 47,000 deliveries (a success rate of 31 per cent)[2] with 61,564 infants. Over 40 per cent were twins or higher-order multiples. Over one-third were small or premature at birth, and many died as a result. These scientists also emphasise that premature and

---

1   This was published in 2013 – it took three years to collate and interpret the figures.

2   This success rate is about 6 per cent higher than in the UK, and almost certainly largely achieved as a result of the risky strategy of putting more embryos back into the uterus in many treatments, as only around 5 per cent of women had a single embryo transferred; many had three or more.

small infants, indeed even twins, are more common after IVF even when single embryos are transferred.

In the UK, the HFEA stipulates limiting the number of embryos transferred simultaneously. Not unreasonably, after years of infertility many infertile women are only too ready to risk a multiple birth, particularly with the rising costs of treatment. While twins may not present too many problems, triplets are difficult to deal with and quadruplets can be disastrous. Even if a twin only spends one month in a premature baby unit after birth (at a cost of around £2,500 a day to the taxpayer) the risk of having an abnormal baby with brain damage, or just bringing up so many babies at once, places massive strains on families.

Humans are not built to carry more than one child at a time, and every risk of childbirth is increased by twins. First, a mother's health can suffer. Obstetric haemorrhage, breech presentation, stillbirth, Caesarean section and diabetes, are particularly common. Triplets hardly ever go to term if they survive pregnancy at all. Most are born 6–8 weeks prematurely. Caesarean section is usually needed and most of these babies require intensive care for several weeks in incubators.

Multiple birth, though often welcomed by infertile parents, remains a major source of concern about IVF. Until we have better methods for assessing the viability of each embryo (see page 90), a policy of single embryo transfer, together with cheaper freezing of all spare embryos seems truly necessary. Not all clinics are sufficiently scrupulous in ensuring that their multiple embryo transfer rate is minimised and patients gamble by having more than one embryo transferred.

Long-term risks of abnormality

Whilst the risk of an abnormal baby after IVF is fairly small (apart from the issues related to multiple birth), there may be a longer-term risk. For example, IVF babies are often tiny and a really low birth weight – say less than 2kg (5½lb) – is associated with disease in later life. High blood pressure, heart problems, stroke and osteoporosis are more likely when an underweight baby reaches 50 or 60 years old. There is increasing evidence that the environment in the womb, at conception and afterwards, affects how a person's genes work as they age. This field – so-called epigenetics – is still ill-understood, but there are certain environmental influences during IVF that may be important. Whilst routine IVF is likely to be harmless, even embryo freezing has been shown to be deleterious in some animal species. Whilst this remains controversial, it seems that freezing mouse embryos and thawing them before transfer may be associated with poor cognitive ability in adult life. In my lab, we showed that embryo freezing and thawing temporarily changes how some genes function. This may not be a disease risk but it will be many years before we can be sure that there is no long term risk for some IVF children. Embryo biopsy and sperm microinjection (see ICSI, page 106) may also carry epigenetic risks. Some rodents have changes in their brain in adulthood after these experimental interventions in embryonic life. This is just possibly why autism has been reported more frequently in children conceived after ICSI.

Blastocyst culture may also carry a slight extra risk as there have been some rare reports of changes in imprinted genes of humans afterwards. These genes are particularly important in normal development and, whilst this is not firmly established as definitely a problem, there have been concerns. Rather more children have been born with the rare Beckwith–Wiedemann syndrome (BWS) after prolonged culture to the blastocyst stage. This condition is associated with childhood cancer, and certain congenital abnormalities including obesity, hernias, a large tongue and changes in sugar metabolism.

Ectopic pregnancy

If the Fallopian tubes are damaged or partly blocked, there is an extra risk of ectopic pregnancy. Although IVF embryo transfer bypasses the tubes, ectopics are more common after IVF. When the Fallopian tubes are scarred, the risk of it is just as high after IVF as it is following tubal surgery. Even though an embryo is transferred into the uterus it can move into a Fallopian tube, where it implants. Even when the tubes have been removed surgically, or are blocked where they join the womb, some risk remains because a small part of the tube in the wall of the uterus cannot be excised completely.

Ovarian hyperstimulation (OHSS)

Follicle stimulating hormone (FSH) can cause too many follicles to grow. Sometimes too much FSH has been given or the ovaries are unusually sensitive. This is called hyperstimulation or ovarian hyperstimulation syndrome (OHSS). OHSS is common and usually mild, merely causing some ovarian swelling with abdominal discomfort and a 'bloated' feeling. Occasionally, there is pain low down in the tummy. Mild stimulation makes some women feel unwell for two or three days and occurs in around 8 per cent of cycles. Moderate hyperstimulation causes more discomfort and sometimes general pelvic pain. The abdomen is usually swollen and this degree of hyperstimulation causes tiredness and breathless. In more severe cases there may be general fluid retention, including ankle swelling. Moderate hyperstimulation is uncommon, but it may necessitate a short stay in hospital, usually for observation.

Severe hyperstimulation is rare. This serious side effect causes breathlessness with sufficient accumulation of fluid in the chest or the abdomen to justify surgical drainage. While the fluid is accumulating in the wrong places, an intravenous (IV) drip is often needed to replace fluid in the bloodstream. Loss of fluid into the tissues concentrates the blood, making it thick. Hospital admission is essential because left untreated it can be life-threatening.

Hyperstimulation tends to be worse in pregnant women. It is also true that if you get OHSS after an embryo transfer and are pregnant, the pregnancy is more likely to stick. This is the good news, but if OHSS is anticipated, embryo transfer should be delayed, freezing all embryos until there is no risk of making hyperstimulation worse. Once a new menstrual cycle has commenced, embryo transfer is safe.

Moderate or severe cases of OHSS are mostly preventable with monitoring of ovarian development using ultrasound. There are one or two conditions predisposing to OHSS, particularly polycystic ovary syndrome. Some women just respond very briskly to superovulatory drugs and why this happens is rather unclear. Careful assessment before an IVF treatment cycle may help avoid serious hyperstimulation. If you are prone to hyperstimulation, you may require less FSH and careful surveillance during IVF treatment.

Irregular periods

One complication associated with all drugs given during IVF is that they can make your periods irregular once treatment is finished. Commonly, the first natural period after failed IVF comes unexpectedly. It may be early or late, may last longer than normal and it may be heavier. Sometimes this irregularity continues for three or four months. If problems persist, you should see a gynaecologist as the symptoms may not be due to IVF, but another cause.

Ovarian cancer

There has been considerable worry that fertility drugs may cause ovarian cancer. This anxiety has been fanned by mostly well-meaning but sometimes irresponsible reports that doctors are not telling their patients the truth about the risks. To understand these risks, real or presumed, it is necessary to have some background.

Ovarian cancer is the sixth most common cancer in the world and in the UK, approximately 14 women in every 100,000 are diagnosed with it every year. The incidence of ovarian cancer varies in different countries; it is highest in Switzerland, about 17 cases per 100,000 and only around one per 100,000 in Africa and China. There is a genetic tendency in certain populations. Ovarian cancer seems more common in parts of the world, particularly Scandinavia.

Ovarian cancer is about twice as common in women who have not had children or who are infertile or who delay child-bearing. Women giving birth before the age of 25 are less likely to develop ovarian cancer and roughly speaking, with each five year delay, the chance of getting it increases by about 10 per cent. Some reports suggest that if you have had a miscarriage, your chance of ovarian cancer is higher, but others indicate it is less likely.

Girls who start their periods early are at a slightly greater risk of having ovarian cancer – perhaps one-and-a-half times as much as girls who start menstruation after they are 15 years old. Women who have an early menopause – before 45 years of age – have a lower risk than those who have their menopause after 50. The contraceptive pill seems protective – women who use it for longer than five years reduce their risk of ovarian cancer by around 50 per cent. It is unclear whether women on hormone replacement therapy (HRT) are at greater risk – probably not, although one Greek study suggests that HRT may increase the risk fivefold. One study in Israel by Dr Ron and colleagues, in 1987, suggests that women married to infertile men may have as high as a six-fold chance of developing the disease, but this is unconfirmed. There is some indication that women who don't ovulate are at greatest risk, but in Australia, Dr Venn and his colleagues report that unexplained infertility carries a bigger risk.

The most alarming research was by Dr Whittemore and her colleagues in the USA in 1992. They reported that there appeared to be a considerable increase in ovarian cancer in women who had FSH injections (Pergonal or Humegon) to treat infertility. It caused both anxiety and controversy and still alarms people almost certainly unnecessarily. Since publication, this study has been heavily criticised. The number of women studied was small; there were inadequate clinical controls; there was no proper adjustment to allow for the fact that infertile women were at greater risk anyway; and there was no relation between the amount of FSH or length of time it was given. The study was also based on recall data – that is, women with ovarian cancer were asked to remember whether they had ever taken fertility drugs. This is likely to introduce bias in reporting. There have been several studies since; none confirm the data presented by Dr Whittemore.

The current data is clear. David Healy and his colleagues in Australia followed 30,000 women after IVF, publishing final findings in 2001. They have found no clear link between any of these drugs and cancer of the ovary. Their study included women who have had as many as nine IVF cycles, with no increased risk of cancer. Their research even indicates that women who have IVF may actually live longer than fertile women.

In summary, there is no clear evidence of an increased risk of ovarian cancer in women having IVF treatment or those having fertility injections, compared with women who are infertile. There is some doubt about an increased risk in women who are given these drugs, but who do not become pregnant. It seems that if you are infertile, but get successful treatment using these drugs, your risk of ovarian cancer falls. Possibly women with unexplained infertility are at greater risk as some of these women may have an ovarian abnormality, including a very early form of ovarian pre-cancer, but this must be very uncommon. These drugs have been used in the UK for many thousands of women since the 1960s without evidence here that they cause ovarian cancer.

Risks of other cancers

Cancer of the uterus is more common in women who have not had children but cancer of the cervix is less common. Neither cancer is caused by fertility drugs. Nor is there an increased risk of cancer of the breast after fertility treatment.

Premature menopause

Some women undergoing IVF are worried that drugs that stimulate the ovaries may cause a premature menopause. Their understandable, but totally unfounded, concern is that, because so many eggs are being produced during treatments the ovaries will run out of eggs sooner.

Damage to ovarian vessels or surrounding structures

Although egg collection is done with great care under ultrasound, the surgeon merely looks at an echo on what is effectively a computer screen. A detailed image of the bowel, the bladder or small blood vessels is impossible so the advancing needle may rarely hit one of these structures inadvertently.

Perforation of the bowel happens occasionally during egg collection, but goes unnoticed by patient and doctor alike. It may possibly account for unexplained pain after an egg collection because of inflammation around the perforation site. It is unlikely to be dangerous. However, on rare occasions, patients can develop infection or an ovarian abscess, caused by bacteria from the bowel leaking out of the puncture site. This can make a patient extremely ill and very exceptionally, an open operation may be needed to drain the infection site.

Uncommonly, a blood vessel may be perforated. Excessive bleeding may be noticed when the needle is withdrawn from the vagina. This normally stops and is of no consequence. In 30 years or more of experience of a large number of IVF cycles, I have known only two patients whose bleeding was sufficient to justify intervention to secure the cut artery. This was easily done without serious damage. Both patients recovered completely after blood transfusions.

Feelings during IVF treatment

Regular attendance at hospital, the waiting, travelling and staying away from home are all tiring. Taking drugs, monitoring of follicle growth and the build-up to egg collection cause tension and worry. Women who are working invariably wonder how they are going to cope with their job and what they will tell their boss. In fact employers are more forgiving than most women expect. It is also true that it usually possible to cope with work whilst undergoing IVF. Flexibility of hours is helpful, but in reality the only days off that are really necessary are the day of egg collection and the day of transfer. The chance of pregnancy is not improved in women who stop work. The only reason for stopping is simply to reduce stress, which may make you feel better.

Undergoing IVF is like a steeplechase – once on, you cannot get off the horse with ease; there are unexpected and sometimes unpleasant bumps, if not actual falls. Waiting to see if the follicles respond to drugs is a critical hurdle. The egg collection is a major fence and the approach to it is usually a time of anxiety. People are often disappointed because they think they have produced too few eggs. It can be devastating to wake from egg collection to find that only one, or even no egg at all was collected. Then there is the two-day wait to confirm fertilisation. This period is often tense and people frequently feel restless, or have vivid dreams.

Waiting for results
Tension is greatest once the embryo has been put back into the uterus. For most women undergoing IVF this will be the first time they have had the experience of knowing they produced an embryo. Most patients fantasise that they are pregnant once the embryo is transferred; a very difficult emotion, given that nearly 80 per cent of the time a normal menstrual period is just 12 days away. Nearly all women start to believe they feel as if they might be pregnant – or alternatively as if they have lost the pregnancy. These feelings are merely symptomatic of the turmoil of this treatment.

If IVF fails
Once the transfer is done, you suddenly find you have no medical procedures to distract you. Sometimes the period comes late. A delay of a few days is horrible, but if it is as long as a week (perhaps with an equivocal or borderline pregnancy test) the disappointment that follows can be all-consuming. Even after implantation, there is still the risk of miscarriage – a devastating experience in more normal circumstances, but no effort is needed to think how cruel it seems if you are infertile, having experienced an uphill struggle to conceive in the first place. On top of the grief people feel for the loss of their baby, a profound sense of despair can be overwhelming.

Such a loss inevitably brings home the notion of being sterile, with all the attendant feelings of inadequacy, guilt and worthlessness. Recrimination between partners, and patients towards the doctors responsible for their treatment, can be a problem. Some couples may also feel isolated. This latest setback implies loss of hope of taking part in normal social contacts with people of the same age group bringing their children up, and all the talk of babies, children and schools. It is easy to feel jealous and visits to a hospital, where other women attend for antenatal care, may seem unbearable.

A miscarriage after treatment often means grief for the lost pregnancy and this can be followed by depression. I have seen people who temporarily lose all confidence in themselves, who feel lethargic, unable to concentrate or derive any satisfaction from normal pleasures. Loss of appetite, difficulty in sleeping or feeling helpless with the simplest daily tasks can be very disturbing.

But it is worth remembering that I have seen so many people whose relationships with their partner and with friends and relatives are a huge support and valuable comfort. Don't let me mislead you. Many people eventually find IVF an extremely positive experience. Couples often find it far less unpleasant or demanding than they expected. Women frequently find it easier to cope with a subsequent cycle when they know what to expect. Very often infertile couples feel they are doing something definitive that will resolve their problem of infertility, and how they approach it. For so many women and men it is undoubtedly better to have gone through IVF and failed, than not to have attempted it at all. To have undergone this treatment can give a much-needed feeling of resolution. Now that everything possible has been done, it means they have the strength to move on with understanding. There is no longer a such a need to mourn over a great feeling of loss.

Chapter 7: Additions to IVF

There are many ways in which routine IVF can be added to, or improved, including freezing embryos and eggs, different ways of stimulating ovulation and preparing eggs for fertilisation, embryo selection, screening, egg donation and surrogacy.

Embryo freezing

The risk of multiple births has led units to restrict the number of embryos transferred simultaneously to the uterus. Frozen storage of 'spare' embryos, or cryopreservation, is now widely used. In an average IVF cycle around nine or ten eggs are collected and generally some 60 per cent will fertilise. 'Surplus' embryos can be preserved by deep freezing. A lucky IVF patient who becomes pregnant at her first attempt with a single embryo can keep these embryos in storage, and return for a second cycle of treatment some years later, to attempt another pregnancy with a sibling embryo. A less lucky patient whose first embryo transfer does not result in pregnancy can then use a frozen embryo for a subsequent treatment. In both situations, this avoids the need to go through a full IVF treatment cycle with ovarian stimulation; hence is cheaper than an IVF cycle started from scratch[1]. Frozen embryos can also be donated to other infertile couples with the approval of the genetic parents, or they may be used to research embryo development or improved infertility treatments. Cryopreservation can also be used to preserve embryos from women who have diseases such as cancer or leukaemia, and who are being treated with radiation and/or chemotherapy that may make them sterile.

---

1   Frozen embryo replacement does not save as much money as it should do, largely because clinics charge what I feel are exorbitant annual fees for storage. To date the HFEA has done nothing to regulate this exploitation.

Embryo storage

At very low temperatures (below -196°C), much colder than a domestic deep freeze, the degradation and decay of all tissues slows dramatically. At such low temperatures a live embryo can be held in suspended animation for many years. Liquid nitrogen, with a freezing point of -196°C, is convenient. At room temperature it is an inert, safe gas comprising 80 per cent of the air we breathe, so it also has the advantage of being cheap. All plant and animal cells contain water and if frozen, ice crystals will form inside them. Ice crystals in an embryo will cause damage so 'antifreeze' or cryoprotectants such as glycerol are used. Embryos are bathed in a solution containing cryoprotectants, removing of most of the water in the cells. The technology has been improved by the use of specially designed freezing machines, programmed by computers. Embryos are cooled at a slow, controlled rate, which also helps reduce damage.

Early experiments

Dr David Whittingham researched slow freezing in the 1970s using mouse embryos. Because they contain different amounts of water, embryos from different species require different rates of cooling and thawing. Eggs and sperm, and ovarian and testicular tissue, all need different recipes for the best storage. Dr Whittingham kept frozen embryos for 40 years. He has removed frozen mouse embryos from storage at five-yearly intervals, thawed them and put them into the uterus of a recipient mouse. His mice subsequently gave birth quite normally. It should be theoretically possible to keep frozen mouse embryos for several hundred years without damage.

Is cryopreservation safe?

Freezing human embryos should be just as successful, but doing this in humans is a bold jump. Human embryos are somewhat less likely to produce a pregnancy after freezing. Freezing any tissue may cause subtle changes and that lovely chef, Heston Blumenthal, agrees with me that frozen food tastes 'different'[2]. Generally speaking, however, human

---

2 It was Heston Blumenthal who pointed out that liquid nitrogen produced pretty nice ice-cream too. He put nitrogen-scrambled egg and bacon ice-cream and nitrogen-poached aperitifs on his menu at his restaurant, The Fat Duck.

embryos seem about only as likely to produce a baby as those transferred fresh (see page 59) so freezing may be having some adverse effect.

We can see microscopic damage occasionally after slow freezing. Often what was, for example, an eight-cell embryo before freezing, may frequently show that some cells are dying, missing or fragmented after thawing. Of course, several thousand normal babies have been born after embryo freezing in spite of such damage, and there is no evidence at all of any increase in fetal abnormality. But we cannot say with absolute certainty what problems may become apparent as some of these children grow up.

One concern is that freezing needs cryoprotectants. There are various compounds: one is sucrose, and another dimethylsulphoxide (DMSO). The latter is a powerful solvent that penetrates cell walls very quickly, but it is also a potential mutagen, which means that in high doses has been associated with changes in the DNA. Such effects could go unnoticed until these children are middle-aged adults. Embryologists have occasionally reported seeing visible damage to the cell nucleus after freezing or thawing and have reported seeing some DNA being excluded from the nucleus and lying outside it during freezing procedures, which is worrying.

Freezing with vitrification
A new process called vitrification has been developed when embryos are immersed in a concentrated solution of cryoprotectants and frozen quickly. Any fluid such as water becomes viscous, like syrup, and sharp ice crystals, which might damage the cells or its membranes, do not form. Vitrification gives better results for freezing many cells, including sperm, eggs and possibly embryos.

It is difficult to prove that any form of cell freezing is completely safe. Years ago, some French scientists, headed by Dr Duliost, examined the long-term effect of freezing the embryos from mice. They compared adult mice that had been frozen as embryos, with mice that had not been cryopreserved during embryo growth, reporting some unexpected differences. Mice from frozen embryos tended to grow fatter in old age, and they had changes in their jaw structure. Behavioural testing revealed that these mice were also often different. It is difficult to know what to make of this. The issue is whether the environment required by embryo freezing adversely affects the way genes subsequently work – a so-called epigenetic effect. Unfortunately, a number of scientists wrote very dismissively of the suggestion that freezing is potentially risky, but as far as I am aware, few researchers who are critical of Duliost's findings have yet repeated the work. However, in 2013, Drs Marta Riesco and Vanesa Robles from Spain published experiments with zebrafish[3] – a species widely used in research because their embryos are easily obtained and develop rapidly. Some genes, including those found in humans, showed altered function after freezing and thawing.

Effects of vitrification

Freezing by vitrification is said to be safer. This seems true in the short-term; certainly more embryos survive. The long-term effects may be different. When mouse blastocysts are frozen there may be fewer cells present after thawing and blastocysts may contain reduced numbers of cells which are less likely to be viable. There are other reported effects. Dr Chatzimeletiou's team from Thessaloniki showed vitrification of human blastocysts affects the way chromosomes line up during cell division. A worrying report by Dr Kader in Cleveland, Ohio, showed that vitrification induces DNA damage in mouse blastocysts. Dr Fabian from Denmark has reported that DNA in pig blastocysts may become broken and fragmented. In 2011, Dr Stinshoff from Hanover, Germany, showed that cow blastocysts showed changes in gene function after vitrification. Finally, it is difficult to know what to make of a report from Taiwan by Dr Lin, who reports that considerably more males were born after transfer of thawed vitrified blastocysts in their clinic. The fact remains that although vitrification is widely regarded now as the best and safest process, its potential effect on gene function is poorly understood.

---

3   I have always felt rather sorry for these stripy little tropical fish that thrive in aquaria filled with fresh water. They are translucent and, to a certain extent, transparent so you can see right through them with their internal organs quite apparent. They have no privacy.

If freezing did occasionally cause mutation or changes in how a gene worked, the effect would be unlikely to show up during infancy. Like most epigenetic changes, such problems usually manifest themselves later in life. For example, it is possible that what we do to embryos could predispose to the development cancers or infertility. It is salutary that it was 50 years before we realised that exposure to X-rays during pregnancy increased the chance of offspring developing leukaemia later. This does not mean that embryo freezing causes cancer or infertility, just that it should still be considered cautiously. Until many children produced from frozen embryos are fully grown we need to be vigilant. At present I would prefer to use embryo freezing when there are no obvious alternatives (see below). But these limitations on embryo freezing are a 'counsel of perfection'. The pressure on clinics and their patients to do everything to avoid multiple pregnancy is great. In the absence of clear evidence that embryo freezing is harmful, this compromise seems inevitable.

Egg freezing

In the last ten years, there has been huge interest in helping older women preserve their fertility as more women are leaving child-bearing

WHEN IS FREEZING JUSTIFIED?

The following are situations when freezing is clearly justified:

- For women over 40 years old who cannot wait for another IVF attempt if the first one fails.
- For women needing cancer treatment that may make them infertile.
- When a woman becomes ill during IVF (for example, after FSH administration or serious hyperstimulation, see page 65) it makes sense to delay embryo transfer.
- For people receiving a donor embryo. A period of quarantine is desirable before the transfer of the embryo to ensure that the donor is free from serious disease like AIDS.

later. A great advance in our society has been the accent on improving the education and skills of women so that they can compete with men equally. In the UK, the average age of a woman with her first pregnancy is now over 30 years old. As more women delay pregnancy until their late thirties or forties, many find themselves infertile. Not unsurprisingly, they worry about being left childless so many consider storing their own eggs in the deep freeze until they find their ideal partner. Attempts at storing human eggs by freezing has had such publicity that many IVF clinics enjoy a substantial market.

There are other indications. Egg storage for women having cancer therapy that may cause early menopause is one example. Another is egg donation as there is a great demand for donor eggs and eggs from patients who have successfully completed treatment. The embryos can easily be stored in liquid nitrogen and fertilised later for transfer to women who have no other chance of a child.

Research and development

Dr Chen in Singapore was responsible for the first baby born after egg freezing in 1987. He used a process devised for embryo cryopreservation by the brilliant Alan Trounson in Australia. But freezing eggs seemed risky as animal research had indicated critical problems. Limited experiments in mouse eggs showed that freezing and thawing could disrupt the genetic material. Dr Peter Braude and Dr Martyn Johnson (now both professors) did important experiments suggesting that some offspring might be born with defects. So, until relatively recently, egg freezing was regarded as too risky. But it seems that the serious genetic effects these professors reported may have been prevented by using a slow cooling procedure or by vitrification.

But freezing eggs can cause unwanted changes. Dr Neelam Potdar in Leicester, made a comprehensive review of all publications about egg freezing. Her team evaluated 21 different studies in over 11,000 human eggs, which showed considerable inconsistencies. There is no doubt that egg freezing is a good deal less successful than wildly optimistic articles in newspapers and women's magazines suggest (or, indeed, the claims made by some clinics). Although very optimistic claims for vitrification are made, it seems only marginally better. In this review, just under 90 per cent of eggs survived thawing, and around 75 per cent were capable of being fertilised. But only 7 per cent of those developing into embryos gave rise to a pregnancy. Approximately 20 per cent of pregnancies ended in miscarriage. I am unconvinced that a 7 per cent success rate would persuade many women that money spent to have this procedure for their advanced age is particularly good value. As to safety, no serious estimate can yet be made as too few births have occurred and those babies have not been followed up for long enough to make a serious assessment. I am not aware of any plans for long-term follow-up so any adverse epigenetic effects may take a long time to be uncovered.

The depressing figures published by Dr Potdar agree with limited data recently obtained from the HFEA. Up to 2012, the most recent year for which there are figures, 2,262 women in the UK have had a total of 20,465 eggs frozen. Only 243 women freezing their eggs or having frozen egg donation have been treated and altogether there have been 253 treatment cycles. There have been 21 pregnancies (around 8 per cent), but the number of live births is not recorded. Given that most of these women were almost certainly relatively young when their eggs were stored, this is not particularly impressive. It does not seem a suitable treatment for older women, because women then generally have eggs of less good quality, and they tend not to respond so well to ovarian stimulation. So those who panic at around the age of 36 or older and who then decide to freeze eggs because they haven't yet found a suitable partner are probably rather over-optimistic.

Why this rather poor success rate? Not enough animal research has been done, but we can learn from studies, for example, in cows. In animal breeding there is a need for these technologies; storing frozen cattle embryos is used to maintain and improve livestock. Consequently, there is more experience amongst those dealing with eggs and embryos of farm animals than with any other mammalian species.

Dr Spirico and his colleagues in Brazil have used the method of vitrification employed in freezing human eggs to evaluate the effect on cows' eggs. Freezing at various stages during egg development showed that thawed vitrified eggs often showed impaired development. They concluded that while the genes in the egg appeared to work normally, freezing caused profound physical damage. The appearances down a microscope clearly showed many cows' eggs had changes in the substance of the cell (the cytoplasm) with some breakup of genetic material. Of course, cows may be particularly susceptible to the risks of freezing because the proportion of water in their eggs is dissimilar to humans.

If egg freezing could be perfected (which seems unlikely in the near future) it would be very valuable. Certainly, it could have advantages over embryo freezing. Freezing embryos can raise ethical difficulties and are hostage to fortune for parents. Should something happen to one or both of them, the disposal of their embryos may raise legal and moral issues. Unfertilised eggs carry much less moral status, and their disposal would presumably be easier. Egg freezing could, paradoxically, also be safer in the long run. This is because after thawing, a frozen embryo is more or less immediately transferred to the uterus, offering little opportunity to check whether it is growing normally. By contrast, a thawed egg has to be fertilised, which in itself is one test of normality. There is the opportunity to observe the subsequent growth of the embryo over several days. If the freeze/thaw process had caused damage, cell division might be disturbed. But most important is that a number of different ways of assessing embryo quality are being developed and it may be possible to check whether freezing is causing damage to chromosomes or genes.

Better drugs to stimulate ovulation

I remain sceptical that any change in drug therapy alone is going to make a huge difference to IVF treatments; possibly the big 'breakthrough' will come when we do not need to give these drugs at all, or find more physiological methods of inducing ovulation. This is one reason why the recent focus on 'mild' IVF is welcome (see overleaf).

One recent compound that just might lead to more 'natural' treatment is Kisspeptin, a protein produced in the brain. The gene responsible for it, KiSS-1, was discovered in 1996, but its relevance for IVF is only just being explored. Interest in KiSS-1 was originally because of its importance in cancer formation; the letters 'SS' indicating that it is a suppressor gene, in other words, it prevents the growth of some cancers. But it now turns out that it has another function. It was discovered in Hershey, Pennsylvania, USA, the town famous for chocolate bars. Hershey's make a confection called a Hershey's Kiss, so the kiss stuck. Kisspeptin seems to be important during puberty and probably ovulation. It is released by cells at the base of the brain, which in turn stimulate the release of hormones that act on the pituitary gland. In particular, it seems to regulate the release of the body's own gonadotrophins, and is sensitive to oestrogen, so its effects may shut down if the ovaries are overstimulated. Some pilot work has been conducted at Hammersmith Hospital and 53 patients have had an encouraging birth rate. We will have to see whether Kisspeptin, and other brain hormones like it, end up as part of the armamentarium of doctors treating IVF patients. It is intriguing that researchers have recently found Kisspeptin in the cells surrounding eggs in the ovary and also in sperm.

Natural cycle IVF and mild ovarian stimulation

The very first successful IVF treatments cycles were not artificially stimulated except occasionally with the drug clomiphene, which affects the ovary. Clomiphene was not ideal because its anti-oestrogenic properties were thought to cause adverse changes on the lining of the uterus. Giving large doses of gonadotrophins, follicle stimulating hormone (FSH) and luteinising hormone (LH), seemed more efficient as this overrode the control of ovarian function, persuading the ovaries to yield many mature eggs. It soon became obvious that blasting the ovaries in this was akin to using a blunderbuss – a crude but effective recipe that worked reasonably effectively.

In the 1980s it became clear that although many eggs could be harvested after large doses of FSH, many of these eggs were not normally matured and had chromosomal and other abnormalities. With my friend and colleague, Professor Stephen Hillier, we lowered the standard dose of FSH substantially. Hillier's understanding of the hormonal control of ovulation during our time together was the major reason for the great success of the IVF programme at Hammersmith Hospital. In 1985, he published a paper describing our earlier success with a 29-year-old woman who, using clomiphene with relatively low doses of FSH, produced just four follicles, each containing an egg. Each egg fertilised and four embryos were obtained. In those days the risks of multiple pregnancy were not fully understood and we transferred all four embryos achieving the world's first quadruplet pregnancy after IVF. These babies survived after delivery by Caesarean section. What was instructive was that the modified dose of gonadotrophins led to high-quality eggs (and therefore embryos) and four normal babies. However, the 'achievement' of a quadruplet pregnancy opened our eyes to the risks of multiple embryo transfer and after this we reduced the number of embryos we transferred.

Nonetheless, high-dose FSH treatment inevitably became the choice of most IVF clinics worldwide – it worked and enough normal eggs could be produced, which led to a reasonable chance of successful pregnancy. Refinements, like the use of drugs to suppress the pituitary function (down-regulation with Buserelin, see page 53) made it easier to use large doses of FSH more efficiently and to time egg collection better. But this approach, still in general use, is even more unnatural. Frankly, market forces have tended to dominate IVF treatment in recent years and FSH use has been sufficiently successful for few researchers to look for more natural approaches.

Many eggs are not viable after heavy stimulation, and some women do not respond well to gonadotrophins. Consequently, there has been a resurgence of interest in 'natural cycle IVF'. For many years this has not received enough serious consideration, but there are now a number of clinics that have quite good experience with minimal stimulation. The advantages are that by avoiding gonadotrophins, the risks of hyperstimulation are largely avoided. Secondly, the drugs used to stimulate ovulation are expensive so there is a reduction of cost. Thirdly, because only one embryo is usually available for transfer, the risk of multiple pregnancy is reduced. And some people, mostly from religious conviction, would rather not be responsible for the unnecessary creation and disposal of human embryos. But against these advantages, the monitoring of follicle development is critical and the demands on the skill of an IVF team are considerable. Success rates with this approach are not as good as with stimulated cycles, but repeated cycles are less demanding.

Quite recently, American authors have reported on success rates for unstimulated IVF. Dr John David Gordon and his colleagues, have only just published the figures in the USA for 2006 and 2007. They record 795 treatment cycles, rather less than 1 per cent of all stimulated IVF cycles in the USA. The total pregnancy rate per cycle was 19.2 per cent with 15.2 per cent live births in women aged less than 35 years old. The birth rate fell off sharply with age, women aged 35–37 having 14.9 per cent live births, and women aged 38–40 having a success rate of 8.7 per cent. Only 2.4 per cent of women aged 41–42 were successful and there were no pregnancies in women over 42. With further experience it may be possible to improve on this significantly lower success rate.

One problem with gonadotrophin-free IVF cycles is that many women ovulate prematurely and the chance of collecting a mature egg is reduced. Many clinicians, like Dr von Wolff and colleagues at the University of Bern, Switzerland, have therefore reverted to that early form of stimulation, the use of clomiphene. They reported the results of treatment in 118 women (average age of 35) treated with 25mg clomiphene from day 7 of their cycle and with a single injection of hCG to induce ovulation. The pregnancy rate was 13 per cent per cycle. If they did not give clomiphene the chance of pregnancy was a bit higher – presumably an effect on the uterine lining. This is clearly a viable treatment even though the success rate is a lot lower than with conventional IVF. Treatment was cheaper and patients merely needed two hospital visits before egg collection. The risk of multiple birth was avoided.

Mild IVF

The term 'mild IVF' has gained slow acceptance amongst some doctors. It is essentially a low-dose regime, aiming to persuade the ovaries to yield eggs of better quality. Mild IVF involves the use of gonadotrophins, in lower doses and for less time than in conventional IVF. Usually, gonadotrophins are started on the day 7 of the menstrual cycle, often after a short treatment with a gonadotrophin-releasing hormone antagonist. Recently, a group of enthusiasts for this approach headed by Dr Bart Fauser from Holland, Dr Nargund from London, Professor Ledger from Sheffield and Dr Tarlatzis from Greece, published a paper 'Mild ovarian stimulation for IVF: 10 years later'[4].

The advantages they claim for mild IVF are that some clinics get results that are almost as good as with conventional, heavy stimulation; that there is less risk and fewer side effects for the patients; that this approach costs less; and that there is a beneficial effect on egg and embryo quality. The disadvantages are unquestionably a lower pregnancy rate, that there are still extreme reactions to gonadotrophins in some patients and the costs are still high.

One impressive paper on mild IVF is by Dr Bodri from Belgium, working in collaboration with colleagues in Japan. For at least 20 years there has been more interest and expertise in Japan in mild IVF than in most developed countries. Over three years, they treated 727 patients with a total of 2,876 cycles. On average each patient underwent four cycles of mild IVF, but some had as many as nine cycles. They mostly used clomiphene with low-dose gonadotrophins, transferring only single embryos. It seems that a number of these patients – close to half of them – received only clomiphene, at least in the first cycle. Because the administration of even low-dose gonadotrophin produced some excess eggs, they used vitrification for a number of embryos. While it is unwise to compare results in Japanese women with, for example,

---

4   One might somewhat uncharitably observe that what they coin 'mild IVF' is very similar to the stimulation regime that Steve Hillier had devised and published 30 years earlier when we retrieved just four eggs from our patient and ended up with quadruplets. It seems a pity, if not a little careless, that Dr Fauser's group do not even bother to quote our paper in their citation list.

Europeans (there are few overweight Japanese patients), the results were impressive. Nearly two-thirds of the women treated had reached the age of 38 at the start of treatment and most had already failed at least one IVF treatment in other clinics.

But though they treated 52 women of 45 or over, some bravely going through nine cycles none over 45 delivered a baby or even became pregnant. Eight out of 202 women between the age of 41 and 44 became pregnant, but sadly none delivered successfully. Although mild IVF has been suggested as an alternative for older women, this excellent Japanese study probably should kill that idea. But these doctors were much more successful with younger women. If we exclude the 254 older women, there were 473 women under 41. The overall live birth rate after one cycle was 17.5 per cent and after two cycles 38 per cent. By three cycles no fewer than 44 per cent had conceived, and after four cycles 48 per cent. Moreover, 65 women underwent nine cycles with two finally achieving a live birth. This study is impressive for several reasons – certainly emphasising that IVF has not been tried properly until three cycles have been completed. It also confirms that single embryo transfer is a viable option to curtail multiple births. I find it interesting for another reason. Some 25 years ago, Kate Hardy and I at Imperial College at Hammersmith suggested that on average only about 18 percent of normal-looking embryos would produce a viable pregnancy and birth. We were criticised for a calculation that seemed on the low side, but these recent figures published by Bodri fit perfectly with our observations.

Although 'mild IVF' is obviously not quite as successful as conventional treatment, the question remains over why it is not used more. Although it avoids expensive drugs, it is not otherwise cheaper, and patients need inconvenient regular hospital visits, with monitoring every two days. Finally, the skill of the embryologists is important and I wonder whether many clinics will have the laboratory expertise to obtain the fine results Dr Bodri reported.

Endometrial scratch

It remains a mystery how the embryo implants into the uterine lining. Even after billions of human conceptions and over five million IVF babies, how the embryo signals its presence in the womb, and womb responds by preparing the environment for implantation is not fully understood. In 1907, a German doctor, Dr Loeb, described an experiment in guinea pigs that was almost totally ignored for the best part of a century. What he called 'nodes' (or knoten) developed after injury artificially made in the uterine lining after sexual activity. In 2003, Dr Ami Barash together with his colleagues from the Kaplan Medical Center in Rehovot in Israel, described a remarkable experiment, which improved implantation in humans after a similar injury. Dr Barash worked for some time in my laboratory at Hammersmith – a more modest, gentle and thoughtful doctor it would be hard to find. On return to Rehovot, he followed 134 randomly selected patients who had failed to get pregnant after an embryo transfer. During the next menstrual cycle before IVF treatment a small tube was introduced into the uterus through the cervix during four separate outpatient appointments. Dr Barash made a tiny injury in the uterine lining by sucking out a tiny portion of the tissue; this so-called endometrial biopsy (see page 39) causes minimal discomfort for a few seconds at worst. Forty-five patients were randomly assigned to have endometrial biopsies; most had already failed four or more IVF treatments. Of these, 30 (67 per cent) conceived, compared with 27 out of 89 (30 per cent) in an untreated control group. Other researchers repeated this study and it seems that in selected patients – particularly those who previously failed IVF an endometrial injury may help.

How does an endometrial injury or 'scratch' produce this effect? A colleague of Dr Barash's, Dr Nava Dekel, from the famous Weizmann Institute, believes that the uterus may become more receptive after injury because of inflammation.

It seems to increase the influx of white blood cells (macrophages and dendritic cells[5]) and these cells stimulate important messages between embryo and uterine lining.

When one works in this bizarre and complex field for long enough one eventually realises that nothing is certain. In 2015, Tracy Wing Yee Yeung and colleagues from Hong Kong, published a randomised controlled trial that failed to reproduce the extraordinarily successful results produced by Dr Barash. They followed 300 patients, of whom two-thirds had not had a previous IVF cycle. In a totally randomised way, 150 otherwise unselected women were sent for endometrial biopsy on one single occasion on day 21 of the preceding menstrual cycle; 150 had no prior treatment. Many of these patients had more than one embryo transferred; 39 of the patients who had a biopsy (26 per cent) delivered a live birth, whilst 48 women in the untreated group (32 per cent) had babies. So there seemed no advantage in the scratch in this entirely unselected group of women.

So, in summary, the early promise of the endometrial scratch remains questionable. The history of IVF is full of examples of initial optimism after exciting new discoveries, followed by a descent to Earth after more realistic appraisal. However, Dr Yeung's study did not identify women who had previously had multiple failures after embryo transfer, so for this group of women, Dr Barash's innovation might be helpful.

In vitro maturation of eggs

Years ago it seemed that maturing eggs outside the body would improve IVF as it might be possible to dispense with the use of expensive stimulatory drugs. To achieve fertilisation, the egg has to be properly matured. Maturation of the egg is a complex process taking place over months (if not years), with a massive spurt during the menstrual cycles before ovulation. The use of injections of FSH is a way

---

5 Dendritic cells are part of the 'white' cell system in the blood. They have a very folded surface that helps them to attach to antigens, which are then tackled and neutralised by other cells in our immune system. They are called dendritic because during development they grow fine branches (dendrites) like a tree.

of inducing that last spurt artificially, to persuade the ovary to produce more mature eggs.

The process of maturation is complex and is under the control of various genes. These need to be activated in a controlled fashion to produce 'good' eggs. Maturation involves augmenting the cells immediately surrounding the egg to provide the nutrients and energy required for development. The egg too, as it matures, starts to initiate its own metabolic processes. Maturation changes the unreceptive egg and makes it receptive to sperm and capable of penetration. It allows the egg to develop a barrier preventing fertilisation by more than one sperm. It means preparing the chromosomes so that they can pair with the chromosomes packaged in the sperm to form a new individual.

Clearly doing this artificially is tricky. But if we could, reproductive medicine would undergo a great revolution. If we understood the maturation process, we could have a method for treating those women who respond poorly to drugs. But it would fundamentally change pretty much all infertility treatment.

An adult woman's ovaries may contain 400,000 eggs, a child far more. All of these eggs are near the surface of the ovary in a thin layer immensely rich in primitive follicles. During a lifetime a few hundred are ovulated – in a society like ours between two or three end up as a child. The rest are wasted. One or two square millimetres of ovarian surface tissue – a piece smaller than the head of a match – will contain perhaps 1,000 eggs. That is enough eggs for the reproductive lifetime of several women – more than enough to complete 300 average families. If we took a tiny piece of ovary, extracted the eggs, stored and matured them, we would improve fertility treatment radically. There would be enough free eggs for donation. We could treat young women who develop cancers, giving them back their eggs after their treatment. We would ameliorate the concerns of women reluctant to get pregnant because of their career, allowing egg storage to avoid the ageing process.

We would also make fertility treatment far cheaper, less involved, and safer. Instead of giving heavy drug treatment to women, we would give a tiny amount of these drugs to the tissue in a glass dish. There would be no ultrasound monitoring, no hormone tests, no risk of hyperstimulation or multiple birth and no side effects or discomfort for women. Eggs matured in the laboratory would simply be fertilised by the partner's sperm and the embryos placed in the uterus by a quick procedure.

How close are we to achieving this? First, it is easy to take pieces of the ovarian surface. Using laparoscopy, surgeons can do it without damage or bleeding. But ovarian tissue could be retrieved on an outpatient basis just by using a needle with some local anaesthetic. And it is easy to store such tissue. Dr Outi Hovatta, in our laboratory at Hammersmith on secondment from Finland, developed simple methods for preserving the ovarian tissue in culture media, and then freezing it. Professors Gosden in Leeds and David Baird from Edinburgh showed it could be functional after thawing. Using transplantation experiments in sheep they proved that fertility could be restored after return of ovarian tissue. Moreover, it is not too difficult to remove the tiny primitive follicles containing eggs from the ovary. In our laboratory Dr Ronit Abir from Israel managed to do this using careful and delicate dissection. Others have done it by dissolving away the unwanted tissue surrounding the follicles with chemicals. And FSH can be given in tiny amounts to ovarian follicles in culture medium allowing them to mature to a limited extent. So it might theoretically be possible to take eggs from the follicles and induce the last stages of the egg maturation process. Eventually we may be in a position to attempt to fertilise eggs treated in this way.

Such an approach will have a radical effect on the availability of IVF. Instead of costing several thousand pounds with drugs, treatment will be easily affordable, costing no more than a few hundred pounds and repeated with little difficulty. All this would give women immense control over their own fertility.

Such technology would represent not just an advance in the treatment of infertility, but would have huge social implications for all of society. Ovarian storage could become a form of family planning. A woman's declining fertility need no longer be an obstacle to her in mapping out her career. A student could store pieces of ovarian tissue while she was at university, then establish herself in her chosen career. Even though she might be in her forties or even fifties, her eggs would be likely to be as fertile as they were when they were first stored 20 years earlier.

Zona drilling and assisted hatching

Zona drilling was first done in 1986 at Hammersmith Hospital, originally as part of a programme to help those couples who carried a genetic disorder (see page 94). A hole was drilled into the zona pellucida, the 'shell' surrounding each egg and a cell extracted for study so that we could analyse the DNA.

When we published early results of zona drilling for genetic diagnosis, some colleagues were surprised that the results of our treatment were so good. In spite of the fact that a cell (or even two cells) had been removed from the embryo, the chance of implantation after drilling a hole in the zona seemed higher than normal. People wondered whether zona drilling gave some clinical advantage. It was supposed that the outer lining of the egg was weakened and the embryo would be helped to hatch, known as 'assisted hatching'. We already believed some eggs (and therefore embryos) were surrounded by a thicker and tougher than average zona. It was presumed that such a zona would not readily break spontaneously as it should five days after fertilisation. Consequently, embryologists started to drill holes in the zona in women who had poor IVF success rates and in eggs presumed to be surrounded by a thick shell.

As with so many reproductive techniques, initial results of assisted hatching were greeted with considerable enthusiasm. However, it was not until 1993 that any controlled trials were done and when they were, drilling holes seemed to make no difference. There was a suspicion that older women had a slightly better chance of success than average. The first group to report this was led by Dr Benjamin Fisch in the Beilinson Hospital, Israel, but with the honesty for which he is well known, he expressed doubts. There probably is little genuine benefit, but some groups occasionally drill holes in the zona in the eggs of women over 40.

Licences for zona drilling

In the UK, the HFEA will not allow zona drilling unless the unit has a specific licence. The HFEA remains unconvinced of its value. This makes me wonder why this regulatory body allows private clinics to charge for what is an entirely experimental treatment with no proven value. Moreover, considering that the HFEA was concerned that drilling could possibly cause micro-organisms like viruses to enter the embryo and cause embryonic abnormalities, their decision seems odd. In my view zona drilling is both harmless and useless.

Non-invasive embryo selection

To reduce the risk of multiple birth, the future of IVF must be to find ways to choose embryos with the best chance of viability and to transfer them singly.

Better chemistry is required

Various tests on embryos in culture have attempted to single out those most likely to implant. One of the first of these was assessment of metabolism. The more energy an embryo uses, the more likely it seems to be growing actively and to be viable. Several hours after fertilisation we placed an embryo in tiny droplets of fluid so small that they could scarcely be seen with the naked eye. Each droplet contained a measured amount of carbohydrate and was isolated under a fine film of oil. Twenty-four hours later each embryo was removed from its droplet and placed in another, freshly prepared one. The original droplet was analysed to see how much carbohydrate was consumed.

Measurements of several hundred embryos in our laboratory consistently showed that more viable embryos used more carbohydrate. One interesting finding was that male embryos seemed, on average, 18 per cent more active than female embryos. Men, it seems, may be more aggressive from the moment of conception. But it turned out that our measurements of consumption were insufficiently discriminatory. There is so much variation in metabolic activity in different embryos. Carbohydrate metabolism is a basic process, and even cells that are dying may absorb considerable amounts.

But this early research may have been useful because it is likely that other metabolic measurements will provide a more accurate test. One promising area we are currently investigating is amino acid metabolism. Amino acids are essential for normal growth and we now have remarkably sensitive methods for detecting just a few molecules of each amino acid. The hope is that by calculating the rate of change of amino acids in culture media, an embryo's potential for development may be gauged.

We can also measure substances called growth factors. Embryonic cells need them to be able to divide. They are chemical messengers that attach themselves to the cell leading to the generation of further messages which control a cell's growth. We found some time ago that embryos require growth factors of various sorts and researchers are assessing which are most important and could be needed to provide the best environment. One further possibility may be to analyse phenomes, or trace molecules, given off by the embryo during cell division. Their presence and the concentration in which they are found, may help our understanding of how the embryo is functioning.

Measuring embryo growth

In the very early days of IVF it was recognised that the rate at which the fertilised egg divided might give clues about its viability. It was hardly rocket science to observe that embryos dividing evenly into similarly-sized cells were likely to be the best embryos to transfer. I remember, as the first Apple Macs came on the market in 1984, using a computer to try to establish an estimate using a simple formula (now rather grandly called an algorhythm – though I am not sure that I knew what that word meant at the time[6]) to predict the likelihood of pregnancy. Until quite recently, there were no really accurate ways of observing the embryo repeatedly during its early development to make more precise observations. Clinics made rather arbitrary decisions whether an individual embryo was developing at an optimal rate and with

6   … and I am still not sure how to spell it.

normal size and shape. A patented device called an Embryoscope has now been manufactured. It is a miniature culture oven with an integrated microscope and camera. It allows time-lapse photography of the developing embryo at regular intervals so the timing of cell division can be recorded. The Embryoscope is effectively a desktop incubator and as such provides a very steady environment in which to observe the embryo; normally, to gain access to a conventional incubator, the door has to be opened and shut and this, of course, may change the environment in which the embryos are being cultured. The Embryoscope is not cheap and, as IVF is now big business, you may be sure that its use is being aggressively marketed.

When this device was first launched in the UK, with the usual media fanfare, one clinic claimed that it had improved their success rate threefold. I remember suggesting to BBC Television News that as this clinic already claimed a 40 per cent IVF success rate, this meant that now over 120 per cent of their patients became pregnant. I said I felt this was curious, but I left the young eager journalist conducting the interview highly impressed. Since then such over-inflated claims have been curtailed, although I believe some clinics are still claiming a 70 per cent pregnancy rate. Of course, as we have seen with every innovation in IVF, wildly optimistic claims are commonly made for improved success that innovation brings; the Embryoscope is certainly no exception.

One early report in 2012 at the Cleveland Clinic, USA, was by Dr Desai who studied 648 embryos from 60 patients transferred after blastocyst culture, having been selected on the basis of their growth rate. Her team reported a 72 per cent pregnancy rate, with 50 per cent of the blastocysts implanting. They emphasise that, by using the Embryoscope, they identified which embryos were most likely to develop. Their results sound encouraging, but this research was on a highly selected population. They only offered the technology to relatively young women and then only those with at least ten good eggs and at least seven embryos. From their results, it seems that they often transferred more than one embryo. Moreover, they report pregnancies rather than the number of live babies, the only measure that interests patients.

Unrandomised trials on selected patients may be encouraging, but give no proof of the effect claimed; this must be done using a randomised controlled trial and, as far as I know, the first was done in Spain. Dr Rubio evaluated results in 843 patients – some having conventional embryo culture in a standard incubator and some in the Embryoscope. All of them had intracytoplasmic sperm injection (see ICSI, page 106) and it isn't clear why they did not use conventional IVF. These patients too, were heavily selected; a number of women with poor chances of success were excluded. The results of this trial are hard to interpret because, rather than reporting the raw data (numbers of patients, number of embryos obtained, number of embryos transferred, numbers of blastocysts transferred, number of pregnancies); they report only percentages and do not report the number of live births. These criticisms may seem nit-picking, but this information is vital for serious appraisal of the value of the Embryoscope. The trial showed a modest improvement in pregnancy rate (about 6 per cent) with the Embryoscope, and a decreased miscarriage rate.

Dr Kirkegaard from Denmark has thrown considerable doubt on the value of the methodology that the Embryoscope uses. They analysed, retrospectively, the implantation rate in 1,519 embryos where they knew the clinical outcome and evaluated their development using the measurements suggested by the Embryoscope. Their study showed that a number of perfectly viable embryos would have been discarded had this instrument been relied upon. Another study by Christian Ottolini and colleagues from the UK and Italy, also questions the value of Embryoscopes, stating that this machine was not greatly helpful in selecting abnormal embryos.

These equivocal results indicate that more trials are needed. This, of course, does not stop clinics that have invested in an Embryoscope from making exaggerated claims. One clinic declares on its website 'The cost to use the Embryoscope as part of your IVF/ICSI cycle is £650. We have purposely aimed to keep the cost of this new time-lapse technology as low as we can, to ensure as many patients as possible can benefit.' Another clinic is rather more modest in its assessment (and charges a lot less – namely £360): 'Embryoscope monitoring is a popular option that is being rapidly adopted by several IVF clinics. At this clinic, so far, 42 patients have used the Embryoscope, with 22 having a positive pregnancy test.'

Embryoscope users across the world collectively estimate that it provides an increase in pregnancy chances of about 5–10 per cent for the 'average' patient attending an IVF clinic. Clearly this may differ depending on individual circumstances and it is still too early to provide robust evidence on outcome, but it might lead to substantial increases in success in women having IVF.

Invasive methods for embryo selection

Our work on the detection of genetic disease led to methods of taking a cell away from the embryo two or three days after fertilisation and analysing the DNA (see page 89). Mutations could be identified and also abnormalities of chromosomes. Unlike most animals, humans produce many embryos with chromosomal abnormalities, that are usually incompatible with survival. Many investigators have tried to assess embryo quality by taking an embryonic cell for analysis if an earlier IVF cycle has failed. This analysis, called preimplantation genetic screening, or PGS, is an attempt to select the 'best' embryos for transfer.

Some clinics attempt PGS on the second or third day of embryo growth and others at the blastocyst stage, usually taking several cells from those which will develop into the placenta. At the preimplantation stage the embryo only has eight cells, so usually only one cell is removed. As a blastocyst may have as many as 160 cells, a greater number can be taken for analysis, giving more accurate diagnosis. DNA or chromosome analysis on single cells requires a high level of sophisticated laboratory preparation and analysis.

It's a very familiar story. As with all new IVF techniques, initial reports were highly optimistic, suggesting that after PGS at either of these stages, pregnancy rates could be doubled. The longer tale is a lot less convincing and it now seems that, even in older women who are most likely to have embryos with chromosomal defects, the value of PGS is dubious. Many private clinics continue to sell PGS to many of their customers, but the published results are discouraging.

As with all medical treatments, it is the randomised controlled trial that is the 'gold standard', and it turns out that these trials do not give much evidence supporting the use of PGS. Certainly more randomised trials are needed because the latest molecular techniques are able to assess the whole genome, and not just individual chromosomes. This may be more helpful. Techniques range from counting all the chromosomes in cells taken from the embryo using a variety of sophisticated methods, to looking at individual changes in the embryonic DNA. So-called 'next-generation sequencing' (NGS), when the entire genome of the embryo can be assessed, is being offered, but it is unclear whether its use really improves embryo selection. One problem is the cost of these procedures and the complexity of the equipment needed. Another is that human embryos are frequently mosaic – that is to say that individual cells taken from an embryo may have abnormalities that the cells left behind do not have. This may lead to perfectly healthy embryos being discarded. Alternatively, the biopsied cells may be normal, but the major part of the embryo that remains has serious chromosomal abnormalities. Until more randomised trials are completed, these issues cannot be resolved.

Improvements in culture media

It seems human embryos obtained after IVF grow more slowly than after natural fertilisation in the Fallopian tube. This is difficult to prove because it is extraordinarily difficult to get access to naturally fertilised human eggs. Some elegant work by Professor Horacio Croxatto in Chile, in the Catholic University of Santiago, was helpful. Patients undergoing routine operations for female sterilisation were asked to have sex without contraception at varying intervals before their surgery. At the sterilisation operation Dr Croxatto flushed out the Fallopian tube and uterus with culture medium[7]. On examination Professor Croxatto

---

7   He obtained ethics committee approval. What a remarkable experiment at a Catholic university!

found that embryos, fertilised naturally were, on average, about one day further advanced in development than we see in IVF media at the same age. Most embryos that continued to develop had become blastocysts by the time they reached the uterine cavity – 96–110 hours after ovulation, or around four days, rather than at five days as we see after IVF.

In most IVF clinics any single embryo transferred to the uterus on the second day after fertilisation has about a 15–25 per cent chance of becoming a baby; in some clinics, where extra care is taken over laboratory techniques, the odds are slightly higher. This variation in the success provides some evidence that the artificial conditions in which embryos are kept are crucial.

Embryos may also have a reduced chance of survival if grown for more than three days in culture media outside the body. Even after culture in the best laboratories, the chance of a four- or five-day-old embryo grown in vitro becoming a baby after transfer is around 30–50 percent. By comparison, Dr Buster's work in California in 1985, was interesting. He collected naturally fertilised human blastocysts from women who had recently had sex, by uterine flushing[8], and transferred them to the uterus of women wishing to adopt an embryo. The pregnancy rate was 60 per cent. Similar results were obtained by Dr Formigli, in Italy, some years later.

Dr Kate Hardy, at Hammersmith Hospital, has shown that IVF embryos often have fewer cells in them than embryos that have grown naturally. Her studies also showed many defects in human IVF embryos. Dying cells are common, and the proteins controlling messages between one cell and the next – the gap junctions – are often deranged. Dr Hardy showed that the cells of many embryos also have abnormalities of their nuclei, and there are more chromosomal abnormalities than one might expect. Of course, some of these observations may be due to fertilisation of abnormal eggs – possibly the massive doses of

---

8 I remember the storm of criticism Dr Buster caused when he announced this experiment at a meeting in Los Angeles. I don't recall now whether he submitted this procedure to an ethics committee.

stimulatory drugs that we give to induce ovulation is deleterious. But these observations may be partly due to inefficiencies in the culture system.

Requirements for embryo development

The correct amount of carbohydrate may promote embryo development and the wrong concentration may inhibit it. We still do not know what is ideal for human embryos, but it is likely that the requirements change during development. It seems that the carbohydrate, pyruvate, is needed for the first two days, but after that glucose is required. It is now agreed that the culture media needs changing depending on the stage of the embryo's development to achieve the blastocyst stage.

Embryos also need amino acids, the building blocks from which our various proteins are made. There are 20 common different amino acids. Perhaps one of the most neglected is glutamine, which some embryos seem to need for best growth. This requirement varies not merely between different animal species, but even between different strains of the same species. Most mouse embryos, for example, need it, although there are some strains of laboratory mice whose embryos develop normally when it is absent. There is also a whole range of other compounds, including inorganic metals and various salts, which should be tested to see if this improves IVF success.

Dr Antony Lighten, one of our PhD students at Hammersmith (now a consultant in Australia), worked on growth factors similar in chemical structure to insulin. The action of insulin in adults is very well known as without it an individual develops diabetes. In early embryos, insulin plays a different role. It acts within the cells, giving instructions for growth. Dr Lighten studied two molecules very much like insulin – insulin-like growth factor 1 (IGF-1), and insulin-like growth factor 2 (IGF-2). Both stimulate growth and cell division in early development. Dr Lighten's work showed that the human embryo is capable of producing its own IGF-2. So the embryo carries the seeds of its own success. But IGF-1 exists in the Fallopian tube and the uterus. We wondered whether it might help embryonic growth and our initial work showed that when it is given to dividing embryos, the chance of survival doubles and the number of cells increases. When these substances have been added to embryos that are to be transferred, there has been no improvement in pregnancy rate. In any case, to tamper with an embryo before transfer needs caution. Before such experiments are done – even though desperate patients are prepared to try – there must be clear evidence that there is unlikely to be a risk to the developing human.

Blastocyst culture

Originally, embryos were transferred on the second or third day after fertilisation; earlier than an embryo would enter the uterus after natural conception. At that stage it is normally in the Fallopian tube, where the environment is different. So it was presumed that the milieu in the uterus is not ideal. During the first IVF attempts, there was always the thought that the fluid in the uterus might be toxic to early embryos. Clearly, the best time for transfer would be when it is ready to implant. Then the endometrium is most receptive and the blastocyst is naturally formed, around five days after fertilisation.

The first IVF culture systems were inadequate to provide the ideal environment for blastocyst development. Even with modern systems many IVF blastocysts have fewer cells than normal. Theoretically, around 50–60 per cent of blastocysts might develop into a fetus. Few clinics, however, have consistently achieved this so it is worth persisting with research.

The transfer of a single blastocyst reduces the chance of twins; if we could always achieve a 50–60 per cent pregnancy rate with just one blastocyst, there would no justification for transferring more than one embryo in most circumstances. The ideal would be to transfer single embryos in repeated cycles, until pregnancy occurs. The problem, of course, is that repeated cycles are costly and people hope for success at the earliest opportunity.

Blastocyst transfer allows better selection of embryos. By keeping embryos in culture for longer, those showing poor development might be 'weeded out'. Also, assessment of the chemicals that embryos are producing could improve information about their viability. The minute differences in metabolic activity on the second and third day that we observed in our laboratories are mostly too slight to make a diagnosis between a normal or abnormal embryo with certainty. But on the fifth or sixth day, when there are more cells in the embryo, such measurements may mean better tests.

Immune screening for implantation failure

There has always been a great deal of interest in the function of the human immune system and early pregnancy. The fetus is made of its own proteins, different from those of the mother. So it should really be rejected at conception or shortly afterwards. Why this does not happen is still an important, but largely unanswered question.

Various antibodies are of particular interest – for example, the anticardiolipin antibody and the lupus anticoagulant. Both may be raised in completely disease-free women prone to recurrent miscarriage. One treatment is to give these women daily doses of aspirin. Another treatment, which is more risky, is heparin. Heparin thins the blood, prevents clotting and may promote unwanted bleeding. There is less evidence that heparin is of real value for repeated miscarriage. Some women are also given corticosteroids which suppress the immune response. Steroids such as prednisolone are not without risk and I feel that this 'polypharmacy' is bad medicine, born out of desperation and frustration.

These medicines have been repeatedly tried with equivocal results in recurrent miscarriage. It seemed logical to try them after repeated failure of implantation after embryo transfer because these unfortunate women may be losing a very early baby. But after nearly 30 years of use, there is very little evidence that heparin or steroids really improve the chance of implantation after IVF failure.

Drugs, including aspirin, may seem justified when there is clear evidence that these antibodies are present in abnormal amounts. A trial in collaboration with Professor Lesley Regan at St Mary's Hospital, London, found that aspirin may be somewhat beneficial. Aspirin is relatively harmless, so a trial of this kind has no serious ethical problems.

Actually, the role of the human immune system in infertility and miscarriage has always been highly controversial. There is no doubt that natural immunity protects the genital tract against infection – the vagina, for example, is full of bacteria, but they generally do not cause disease. Although sperm and the developing embryo contain foreign proteins, they are not rejected and it is probable that cells produced by the immune system allow this foreign 'graft' to be tolerated. One group of cells thought to be involved are natural killer cells (NK cells), which may be increased in the cervix and the uterus towards the second half of the menstrual cycle, and during pregnancy. Their increasing numbers may be a response to changes in hormone levels, presumably progesterone and oestrogen. However, data on the numbers of these cells is very incomplete. Some researchers claim that white blood cells from the immune system decrease when there is failed implantation or miscarriage. The thinking appears to be that, without adequate suppression of the immune response, women may be infertile or lose an early pregnancy. Consequently there has been a vogue in some clinics to give drugs that suppress the human immune system where the infertility is unexplained or where there is repeated early pregnancy loss. These powerful drugs[9] are usually given for serious diseases like severe rheumatoid arthritis.

Review of research
Drs Seshadri and Sunkara from Kings College, London, reviewed this subject in 2014. They analysed 22 publications, finding that some studies reported that there were more NK cells in the peripheral blood of infertile women, than in those who were fertile, and they seemed to be raised in some women with recurrent miscarriage. Importantly, these differences were not statistically significant. The studies they cited did not measure cells in the reproductive tract itself. Another problem was that the way the cells were measured was not standardised so comparison is impossible. They conclude by saying that the immune system is so

---

9   I use the word 'powerful' advisedly. Not only can they increase the risk of infection and suppress a woman's blood count, they are occasionally associated with an increased risk of cancer. Moreover, their effect on any developing baby is not known.

complex that measuring NK cells on their own with dubious assays is probably valueless. Consequently they suggest that the treatments that are currently tried are entirely unproven and that much more research is needed, with good randomised trials. But to add to the controversy, Dr David Clark from Canada, is highly critical of their approach. In a recent article[10], he argues that randomised trials are not always the best way of testing these treatments. I disagree. The problem is that the history of reproductive medicine is littered with examples of false hopes raised by failure to use proper statistical analysis. So for the moment I feel that the evidence to treat 'failed implantation', 'unexplained infertility' and recurrent miscarriage with dangerous drugs is unjustified. Suppression of the immune response must be seen only as a research procedure.

Egg donation

Total inability to produce eggs is not rare. A surprising number of young women – several thousand in the UK – suffer a premature menopause. Their ovaries do not make follicles or oestrogen. These unfortunate women, as well as being sterile, generally need hormone replacement therapy (HRT). This distressing condition, mostly of unknown cause, can strike before the age of 20. Many afflicted young women feel that they are not properly female. Until IVF, there was no treatment for these women. Egg donation, first successfully done by Alan Trounson's group in 1984 in Monash University, Melbourne, Australia, proved revolutionary. It was possible for these women to carry a baby and treatment was surprisingly successful.

Finding egg donors has been difficult. They have to go through the IVF process, having their ovaries stimulated, and then egg collection. No matter how altruistic, this is demanding. Once eggs are obtained, they can be fertilised with the sperm of the recipient's partner and any embryos transferred to her uterus. Because most women who cannot produce eggs are producing insufficient oestrogen, they are given hormones to stimulate the uterine lining to enable an embryo to implant. HRT may be needed until pregnancy is established, thereafter,

---

10 'Popular Myths in Reproductive Immunology', *J Reprod. Immun.*, 104–5:54–62, 2014

the developing pregnancy provides sufficient hormones to ensure its safe development.

Unlike donor insemination (see page 125), egg donation involves both partners in any resulting pregnancy because the husband is providing half the genetic material. Though the infertile woman is not the genetic mother of her child, she nurtures it from conception, carrying it within her own body and, most importantly, gives birth to it.

Indications for egg donation

Egg donation is chiefly used for women whose own ovaries are not producing eggs. Apart from women entering an early menopause or those in the older age group with poor ovarian reserve, other situations in which egg donation may be appropriate are:

- If a woman's own eggs have repeatedly failed to fertilise during IVF the presumption is that they have an abnormality preventing fertilisation.
- When the ovaries respond very badly to ovarian stimulation during IVF or eggs cannot be collected because of scar tissue or ovarian cysts.
- When a woman has no ovarian tissue perhaps because of previous surgery or congenital disease.
- If there is serious genetic disease in a woman's family which might be inherited by her babies. If the defect is undetectable during IVF or pregnancy, egg donation may help her to have an unaffected child.
- If cancer treatment has killed the eggs in the ovaries. The ovaries may recover after treatment; if not, donor eggs may be valuable.

The procedure

Many women who need donor eggs don't have periods, unless on HRT. This means that their endometrium, the uterine lining, is very thin. Even if an embryo is transferred, implantation may not occur. For egg donation to work, it may be necessary to stimulate the uterus. Oestrogen and progesterone are given in a cyclical fashion, creating an artificial menstrual cycle. Donor eggs are then fertilised with the partner's sperm and embryos are transferred to the recipient's artificially stimulated uterus. Because a donor often produces more than one viable eggs, they may donate to more than one recipient simultaneously.

What is the success rate?

Oddly, egg donation cycles are often more successful than routine IVF. In selected patients donor cycles can double the usual IVF pregnancy rate partly because the donors are usually under the age of 35. As a woman ages, more of her eggs seem to develop genetic defects when they mature. Eggs from younger women fertilise more readily and produce embryos that are much more likely to implant. Miscarriage and conditions like Down's syndrome are therefore slightly less common after egg donation.

Egg donation is may be so successful because recipients are not exposed to the drugs used to stimulate the ovaries. During routine IVF these drugs may have adverse effects on the uterus and its lining. Then the ovaries may produce 3–10 times the normal amount of oestrogen. This gets into the bloodstream, where it could result in the uterine lining becoming less receptive to the embryo. In an egg donation cycle, the recipient of the fertilised eggs is not exposed in this way, and is given the right amount of hormone to encourage best uterine development.

Recipients who are totally menopausal and not menstruating may have a better chance of pregnancy with egg donation than women with active ovaries. Donation in younger recipients may be more difficult because of the need to control timing of endometrial development.

Egg donors

Many women seek donated eggs, but there is a great shortage. Few women wish to be donors; hardly surprising given the commitment needed. Apart any psychological and social issues, these factors include:

- Donors need blood tests and possibly genetic screening. They will be tested for infections such as hepatitis or HIV.
- Donors receive the drugs usually given during an IVF cycle. They need monitoring and hospital visits and an operation to collect eggs. This is daunting, especially for women who are bringing up young children.
- In spite of careful supervision fertility drugs may cause hyperstimulation (see page 65).
- Most importantly, donors offer their unique heritage, giving life to a child over whom they have no influence or knowledge.

Embryo donation

A number of embryos, stored after successful IVF treatment, are preserved in liquid nitrogen banks. If the genetic parents have no further need, these embryos can, with consent, be donated to infertile couples. Embryo donation has been described as a form of 'adoption in utero' and it does mean that the recipient gives birth to her 'adopted' child, nurturing it from its earliest days.

Embryo donation is not common; most parents with spare embryos prefer not to donate. By regulation, embryos may not be kept longer than ten years, so most embryos that might be used for another couple's treatment are destroyed at the conclusion of this time limit.

Embryo donation is technically similar to egg donation. It involves careful cycle timing and the uterine lining may need priming with drugs.

Surrogacy

Some women have had their womb removed because of disease and others may have a severely damaged uterus, perhaps because of previous infection of its lining or a severe congenital defect. A girl may be born with a rare, congenitally deformed uterus that is so abnormal that pregnancy is very unlikely. In such cases, IVF is generally futile, and the solution for such patients may be for another woman, possibly a friend, to bear their baby.

Requests for surrogacy are very rare because they are fraught with risk for all concerned. A great deal of careful advice, assessment and counselling is needed. There are also considerable dangers, not least of a tug-of-war between the surrogate mother and the donating parents.

There are two kinds of surrogacy. The surrogate mother's own eggs may be fertilised naturally after artificial insemination from the adopting male partner. In its most primitive form, this obviously does not require medical intervention. It is unknown how often couples enter into this kind of arrangement, but it is clear that it is not that rare. A difficulty will, of course, occur when the child is born. He or she will have to be adopted by the commissioning parents, and a private arrangement may be forced into the open.

Many women with a damaged uterus, or even those born with no uterus, have normal ovaries producing good eggs. An egg can be taken from the ovary of a woman with no uterus and fertilised in vitro. This requires the monitoring associated with IVF and the surrogate needs careful surveillance until the time for transfer into her uterus. Once an embryo has been produced, the surrogate has a transfer to carry the baby, handing it over to the genetic parents for adoption. The social problems concerned with surrogacy, are extensive, but really beyond the scope of this book. Advice may be sought via the Genesis Research Trust website.

Chapter 8: IVF for male infertility

It is said that IVF has been the biggest advance in the treatment of infertility during the last century. The biggest impact has certainly been on male infertility. Once, most male infertility was virtually untreatable. Rarely, evidence-based management was possible, yet results were mostly haphazard. IVF has changed that because it allows direct access to the egg, manipulation of the sperm and the egg together, and clear proof of fertilisation.

In the early days of IVF, fertilisation could be somewhat enhanced by placing a single egg in a droplet containing more sperm than would be naturally possible. The greatest development came with the ability to inject sperm directly into the egg, revolutionising treatments. Once the condition with the worst outlook, male infertility, often now has a good prognosis.

Intracytoplasmic sperm injection (ICSI)

In the 1980s, researchers fertilised mice eggs by injecting single sperm into them. After sucking sperm into a glass needle, this was passed through the outer shell (zona) of the egg and into its substance (the cytoplasm) – intracytoplasmic sperm injection (ICSI). Initially it was considered dangerous because it was feared that it might cause genetic damage to the egg or result in the injection of a harmfully abnormal sperm.

Sub-zonal injection

In the late 1980s, Dr Simon Fishel, at Nottingham University, developed a technique in humans that involved injecting sperm just under the egg's outer shell. He understood that from here less mobile sperm might penetrate the cytoplasm on their own. This was based on the observation that poorly motile sperm could enter an egg if the harder zona had been damaged first. Dr Fishel called this 'sub-zonal sperm injection' or SUZI (I am not sure what the 'U' stands for), feeling this would be safer than injection directly into the egg itself. This might avoid its disruption and the 'best' sperm would still be selected. But he ran into difficulties with the great and good of the HFEA and this authority remarkably refused a licence for a pilot project in the UK. Dr Fishel felt he had quite enough evidence to prove the safety of what he intended and he continued his experiments in Italy[1]. Soon, many once-despairing Italian couples were giving birth to completely normal babies, and couples with a sperm problem in the UK had to travel an inconvenient distance for treatment.

ICSI's early successes
SUZI was eventually superseded, but we should remember that Dr Fishel's work certainly influenced what followed, the subsequent technique of ICSI. This was the much more invasive treatment originally tried in mice. It soon became clear that it was more successful than SUZI and needed just one sperm for each egg. Early worries about genetic damage were assuaged when the first children were born. Those possibly most responsible for the successful development of ICSI were the Brussels team led by Professor André van Steirteghem. ICSI is often useful even when only a tiny number of sperm are available. They may not need to be capable of movement or fully mature, so many couples who previously could only conceive using donor semen now have hope.

The process
A human egg is thinner than a human hair and invisible. When taken from the ovary, it is surrounded by two or three million sticky 'helper' cells, which provide essential nutrients. These are first removed. Once cleaned, the egg is immobilised so that the zona can be penetrated.

ICSI requires delicate manipulation with fine instruments. The

---

1   It is easy to forget how the HFEA, in its wisdom, has often led the world – in this case, the banning of highly successful techniques to treat male infertility.

injection pipette is marginally wider than the diameter of a tiny sperm and is held in micromanipulators allowing very precise movements. To avoid even the slightest extraneous vibration, the microscope and micromanipulators are mounted on an isolated table cushioned by shock absorbers on a solid floor. Sperm normally move fast so catching them in a pipette is tricky. A viscous fluid is introduced which controls their exuberance – somewhat like wading through treacle. Thereafter, the sperm's tail can then be crushed with the end of a pipette. Once immobilised, they can be sucked into the tip of the fine glass tube.

A sudden controlled movement is needed to penetrate the egg, breaking through the zona, and the membrane surrounding the substance of the egg. The nucleus is left undamaged, and care is taken not to go through the egg and penetrate the opposite side. Injection of the sperm head must be gentle and the whole process usually takes several minutes. If there are many eggs, the procedure can take over an hour, so ICSI is quite labour intensive.

ICSI requires experienced embryologists who need much practice before getting good results. It is easy to damage the egg and there is skill in picking up sperm free from obvious defects. A worry has always been that some sperm with undetected abnormalities may be used. Most defective sperm, even when the fault is not obvious, are incapable of producing an embryo. Once ICSI is completed, the eggs are cultured as in standard IVF.

When is ICSI suitable?

ICSI is indicated for men with fewer than, say, 100,000 sperm available or perhaps when there are sperm with inadequate movement. However, when only a very few are normal, ICSI may be unsuitable. It can also be used when high levels of sperm antibodies are present if routine sperm washing is ineffective. ICSI is also valuable after repeated fertilisation failure during a previous IVF cycle. Some patients having preimplantation screening for genetic defects are usually treated by ICSI.

Results of ICSI

The team in Brussels reported a study using nearly 75,000 eggs. Nine per cent of their eggs were damaged by the injection and not used. Approximately 72 per cent of ICSI injections caused successful fertilisation. These figures, years ago, have stood the test of time. These results were remarkable considering the Belgian doctors were using abnormal semen. After all, in most routine IVF programmes only 50–70 per cent of eggs fertilise 'naturally' when the sperm are mostly normal. Abnormalities of fertilisation occurred in about 5 per cent of injections and they could transfer at least one embryo in 90 per cent of the cycles. Nearly 30 per cent resulted in pregnancy. In the UK the HFEA now claims that success rates with ICSI are so close to those using 'natural' fertilisation in routine IVF that they do not record ICSI results separately.

The risks of an abnormal baby with ICSI

There are theoretical risks associated with ICSI. These are:

- That the body's normal sperm screening process is bypassed and an embryologist may inject a genetically abnormal sperm without recognising it.
- That solutions to slow the movement of the sperm may cause genetic damage.
- The injection may disrupt genetic material in the egg cell or introduce extraneous material into the egg.
- Some men needing ICSI have genetic abnormalities they might pass to their offspring.

One might expect, therefore, to see examples of increased risk, but fertilisation rates and embryo formation are actually increased using ICSI. It might also be expected to see reduced pregnancy rates or more miscarriages (both more likely when abnormal embryos are present), but there is no evidence of this is most programmes.

A key observation is the number of babies born with abnormalities. The figures are reassuring. In the UK around 0.6 per cent of babies born after IVF had an abnormality of some kind, and after ICSI this is less than 1 per cent – fewer abnormalities than seen after normal conception in fertile women. Many babies have been born after ICSI worldwide and the incidence of abnormality is just a little higher than in the general population. Yet there is still one unresolved concern. Rather more women than would be expected have requested termination of a pregnancy after ICSI often for major malformations found on antenatal screening. In my view, careful follow-up of all these complex procedures is still justified even though any risk seems minimal.

Screening men before ICSI

To avoid risks to the unborn child, infertile men needing ICSI should be checked for any genetic cause for impaired sperm production. Some men with severely depressed sperm counts may have a chromosomal defect, particularly of the Y chromosome, and others can have a defect elsewhere, for example, a translocation (see page 35). Men with abnormalities of the epididymis or the vas deferens (the tube leading from the epididymis to the prostate gland) may carry the mutation causing cystic fibrosis. If his partner has a similar mutation there is a one in four chance that any child may suffer this disease. There are other genetic diseases too, which are associated with similar abnormalities but they are much less common, and the chance of the female partner having the same defect will be small.

Any man undergoing ICSI, with a low sperm count for reasons that are not clearly established, should have a karyotype (see page 35). Such screening will not totally rule out the transmission of an undetected abnormality, but it avoids most serious chromosomal defects in his offspring.

Epididymal aspiration of sperm

Some infertile men make sperm, but for various reasons they don't get into the ejaculated seminal fluid. A surgical injury or a previous vasectomy are common problems. Occasionally there will be a block somewhere in the epididymis. It was thought that sperm from the epididymis would not be mature and could not fertilise eggs, but ICSI shows otherwise. It is possible to aspirate sperm directly from this very fine duct and use ICSI

WHEN IS EPIDIDYMAL ASPIRATION NEEDED?

Epididymal aspiration of sperm may be indicated when:
- When there is congenital absence of the vas deferens.
- In men who have had a failed reversal of sterilisation.
- When an operation to unblock the ducts of the epididymis has failed, or if the condition is unsuitable for surgery.
- For men who have no sperm in their ejaculate after a hernia repair. These men may have damaged tubing leading from the testicle.

Epididymal aspiration of sperm is often done just before egg collection. Under general anaesthetic the scrotum is incised and the epididymis exposed. Sometimes the whole testicle may be temporarily removed from the scrotum. In most cases of obstruction the epididymis is swollen and dilated. The fine-coiled tube of the epididymis is inspected under a microscope. A tiny incision is made in the tube as far from the testis as possible. Although more sperm are likely to be found close to the testis, once the epididymis is cut it cannot be easily repaired, so the surgeon works back towards the testis in the hope of leaving some tubing for another attempt later if needed. A fine needle is then inserted and suction applied. An embryologist examines the aspirated fluid under a microscope immediately. If no sperm are seen, or if the motility is very poor, the surgeon may make another cut in the tubing, a bit closer to the testis. If no sperm at all are found, the testis will be replaced in its scrotal sac, and the surgeon may explore the opposite side. Once sperm are obtained, eggs are collected. After ICSI any spare sperm can be stored in liquid nitrogen for use if the initial treatment fails. But thawed epididymal sperm are not always as fertile as fresh sperm.

The procedure is similar to testicular biopsy (see page 33) and recovery is usually uneventful. Most clinics now report fertilisation rates after epididymal aspiration which are nearly as good as those after ICSI with ejaculated sperm. Many achieve around a 20 per cent pregnancy rate after embryo transfer. In general, the results of these procedures are better when failure of sperm production is due to blockage of the tubing, rather than when sperm cells are not being produced due to genetic or biochemical disorders, or scarring from infection.

Percutaneous epididymal sperm aspiration

Some surgeons avoid open testicular surgery and try to obtain sperm simply by inserting a needle through the scrotal skin, stabbed directly towards the epididymis – percutaneous epididymal sperm aspiration (PESA). It is possible to retrieve sperm by aspiration in many cases often done with just local anaesthesia. This is like testicular mapping advocated by Dr Turek (see page 34).

It has the advantage of not requiring a formal operation, but it can be painful when the testicle is perforated. Some men experiencing it once are reluctant to undergo a second attempt. Secondly, it does not seem as reliable a method of collecting sperm. The epididymis is a very small structure and, unless it is considerably dilated, it is difficult to identify and introduce the needle. Also, bleeding where the needle enters the testicle can cause postoperative pain. Scarring around the tubes may also make subsequent attempts at sperm aspiration very difficult. An open procedure may be preferred, when a testicular biopsy can be done simultaneously (see page 33).

Testicular sperm aspiration

Sometimes the epididymis is badly scarred or thickened, or the testes are producing only very few sperm. Then the only chance of retrieving sperm may be by direct collection from the tiny tubules of the testis in which the sperm develop. Providing some sperm are being produced, it may be possible to retrieve sufficient for ICSI. This procedure is like epididymal sperm aspiration (see above) done under general anaesthesia. A small piece of testicular tissue is removed, examined microscopically, and washed with culture fluid to release any sperm. If none are seen, the surgeon may remove another piece of testicular tissue. Tissue can be frozen for later attempts at sperm retrieval. If aspirated sperm are fairly mature, the chances of fertilisation are quite good. This approach can be repeated a limited number of times.

When is testicular aspiration futile?

If a man's FSH levels are high, the testes may have stopped producing sperm and if very raised, there may be total testicular failure (see page 33). Then aspiration unlikely to be successful.

When the testes are very small, soft and shrunken, as they are sometimes with testicular failure, sperm manufacture may have stopped and aspiration is much very unlikely to yield sperm. Testicular biopsy can help the decision to proceed to any form of ICSI. If microscopic examination clearly shows that no sperm are being produced and that there is total testicular failure, testicular aspiration is unlikely to be of benefit. This condition is often called spermatogenesis arrest.

Spermatid injection

Some men do not produce mature sperm but spermatids, immature sperm cells that would normally develop into spermatozoa. Sometimes the testes may produce immature sperm normally, but genes controlling how the sperm mature are altered. Spermatids have been injected into eggs using ICSI. They are classified into two main types – round or elongated spermatids; elongated cells are more mature, and round cells are at a primitive developmental stage.

Fertilisation has occurred after injection of either type of spermatid and in some cases embryos develop. In the UK, the HFEA has not as yet licensed the use of spermatid injections for human treatment, because it is thought that injecting such an immature sperm risks producing an abnormal child. Indeed, some reports indicate that spermatid injections have resulted in babies with serious birth defects. Round spermatid injection (so-called ROS or ROSNI) resulted in a few live births some years ago. But most pregnancies ended in miscarriage and there have been no more successes recently. Injection with more mature elongated spermatids (ELSI) has been more successful, with a fertilisation rate close to 50 per cent in a few centres; the pregnancy rate has been as high as 29 per cent. The total number of live births is not well reported as some clinics overseas often confuse pregnancy rate with live births.

Currently, there are attempts to develop immature sperm cells in culture, but without great improvement in success. Opinion varies as to the value of spermatid injection. Many feel that it is dangerously experimental. For men whose testes are working so poorly, donor insemination is probably simpler and wiser when it is acceptable.

Unnecessary ICSI

Some private clinics use ICSI when it is not really indicated. This may be profitable but in my view, ICSI should not be used unless truly required to achieve fertilisation safely. ICSI seems completely safe but it is foolish to use complex treatments when there are simpler solutions. ICSI is also relatively expensive, hardly surprising, given the cost of the equipment needed, the amount of space required in a laboratory, and the fact it needs considerable time by a trained embryologist. There are a number of alternatives that patients may elect to use when undergoing IVF.

Alternatives to ICSI

There are a number of other options available to men with reduced sperm counts.

Mixing routine IVF with ICSI

In an attempt to avoid ICSI, some patients have elected in the past to have half their eggs treated by 'natural' IVF, hoping to use ICSI as a last resort. Commonly some patients have asked that their eggs are split into two batches and treated by the two separate methods.

When ICSI was first used, the HFEA ruled that patients must not have a naturally fertilised egg transferred at the same time as an ICSI egg. Their reason seemed largely to be so that adequate data on the fate of ICSI embryos could be obtained. If a pregnancy occurred after a 'mixed transfer', they would not know whether pregnancy resulted from natural fertilisation or from ICSI. This was typical of a bureaucratic action by the regulatory authority and the decision ignored an individual's choice. The case was argued with the HFEA for over two years, and eventually they changed their view. But now transferring multiple embryos simultaneously is considered dangerous because of the risks of multiple birth (see page 62) in any case.

Percoll treatments
Some men with reduced sperm counts, but motile sperm, can have the number of good sperm enriched. This can be done by passing the sperm through a filtering medium. A widely used fluid is percoll, a viscous solution that allows the best sperm to be concentrated for subsequent IVF. Once sperm have passed through it, they can be placed in a tiny droplet and concentrated around the egg, giving a greater chance of fertilisation. Since ICSI has been perfected, this technique not often used.

Adjuvants to increase sperm vigour
There are a number of substances which encourage sperm activity. Drugs mixed with sperm may increase the chance of fertilisation. One commonly used substance was Pentoxifylline, another is caffeine. There is no doubt that these can increase motility and possibly the fertilising capacity of sperm. But trials have not clearly demonstrated their effectiveness and very few laboratories now use them.

Donor back-up
Sometimes attempts to enhance fertilisation fail so it can be worth having donor sperm ready as a back-up. This has become difficult to arrange since donor sperm has become scarce. If a donor is to be considered, it is important that arrangements are made in advance of IVF rather than deciding on a donor on the day of egg collection. Some doctors will discourage this if appropriate advice and counselling has not been done.

Whenever donor insemination is considered, it is wise for the couple to have unhurried counselling from an expert, familiar with the associated problems. It is essential to explore the family aspects of sperm donation and to review feelings about this very carefully. Both partners must be satisfied that they are prepared to accept donor sperm.

Once donor back-up is agreed, a suitably matched donor should be found. The stored sperm can then be held in reserve depending on the outcome of sperm aspiration. It must be pointed out that once any sperm have been mixed with the eggs or once ICSI has been undertaken, it is too late to use donor sperm. One way around this is to separate some eggs for ICSI, retaining others for donor insemination. This does, of course, reduce the number of eggs available for treatment.

Emotional aspects of ICSI

Most ICSI is done with ejaculated sperm rather than those taken from the testicle. Even when a woman is completely normal and the problem is entirely with her partner, she has the burden of most of the treatment, including extensive stimulation with drugs, daily monitoring, egg collection, embryo transfer and the anxiety of waiting to see if she is pregnant. She also takes the risks involved. Remarkably, many women prefer this; others find it a considerable strain. Some women feel that it gives them some kind of control over the whole process as many women do everything to protect their man from the consequences of the infertility. This can put considerable strain on a relationship, and some men feel very guilty about the effort that their partner has made, or the risk she undergoes. It is important for these issues to be carefully thrashed out before treatment.

Chapter 9: Other successful treatments for infertility

There are many conditions that cause infertility which, treated appropriately, have a much better chance of success than one or two cycles of IVF. A key issue, as I have already emphasised, is making a diagnosis.

Treatments that encourage ovulation

Drug treatment is by far the most effective therapy when failure to ovulate is causing infertility. Generally speaking, about 80 per cent of younger women who are not ovulating who are treated with pills or injections to stimulate their ovaries, can expect a pregnancy. Women who are over 38, or those who have an incipient menopause, are not nearly as likely to get pregnant, either with drugs, or by using IVF.

Clomiphene treatment

Clomiphene is the standard fertility drug, (usually marketed as Clomid). It has some properties similar to oestrogen and was originally developed in an attempt to find a contraceptive pill that did not have the side effects associated with oestrogens. But early testing in rats resulted in some animals getting pregnant rather too easily, so its future as a contraceptive seemed distinctly dodgy. Indeed, some rats given clomiphene were actually more fertile than normal. Finally, in 1961, Dr Greenblatt in the USA, showed clomiphene helped women who did not ovulate.

Clomiphene is a good first-line treatment; it is cheap, free from major side effects and rarely causes multiple births because it is a weak stimulant. It promotes ovulation by encouraging the natural release of follicle stimulating hormone (FSH) from the pituitary gland, making the ovaries work harder. But, because clomiphene is an anti-oestrogen, it can thicken cervical mucus, making it less penetrable by sperm. It can also interfere with the uterine lining, possibly preventing embryos implanting. Stimulation with clomiphene can cause ovarian cysts so its use needs supervision.

In the late 1990s, an article in *The New England Journal of Medicine* suggested a very slightly increased risk of ovarian cancer in women who had taken clomiphene for long periods. There was no evidence that this was a problem unless a woman had been taking it continuously for over one year at least. It was not associated with other diseases, such as uterine or breast cancer. In any case, this report is dubious because all women who are not fertile or not had children, are already at slightly higher risk of ovarian cancer (see page 66). Responsible medical opinion clearly believes that clomiphene, given for less than a year or so, is totally safe.

Usually one tablet (25–50mg) is taken daily for five days, generally starting on day 1 or 2 of menstruation. If the woman's cycle is much longer than 28 days, clomiphene may be given from day 5 for five days. The dose can be increased if there is no ovulation. Symptoms suggesting ovulation are breast tenderness, mid-cycle abdominal discomfort, vaginal discharge (at ovulation) and more regular periods, but none are conclusive proof of ovulation. Hence tests to check ovulation are needed. Ultrasound is best as it confirms ovulation but can also detect cysts. Blood progesterone level is often measured, but is less reliable because clomiphene can stimulate the production of more than one follicle at the same time, but without ovulation. The combined amounts of progesterone from follicles that have not ovulated can cause a rise in progesterone to apparently ovulatory levels (30nmols or more).

Clomiphene may cause hot flushes. A few women get frequent or irregular periods and if this happens they may need to stop the drug. Cysts are not serious, but if they develop the drug should be stopped to give the ovaries a chance to recover. Some people may feel unwell while taking clomiphene. There are other drugs that can be taken instead, such as tamoxifen or cyclofenil. They tend to be less effective and more expensive.

Clomiphene is usually be discontinued if there is no pregnancy after 6–9 months. There is little value continuing it for more than one year.

Gonadotrophins

Human menopausal gonadotrophin (hMG) and follicle stimulating hormone (FSH), originally marketed as Pergonal or Humegon (see page 54), were the first mixture of these hormones to be used. They are given by injection. FSH is a powerful drug which must be given under close supervision. Usually these drugs are used when clomiphene has failed, but they have a place as an initial treatment, particularly for women not having periods. I should add though, they are much less suitable for anorexic women who are not menstruating, in which case their use can be dangerous. Attention to diet and weight are mandatory in the first instance.

Genetically engineered FSH has now virtually entirely replaced hMG because it is less likely to cause allergic reactions and its effect is more predictable. But these drugs come at a price because the process of developing genetically engineered is so involved. FSH is usually injected daily early in the menstrual cycle until ovulation is imminent – usually 5–10 days later. When ovulation is about to occur, a triggering injection of human chorionic gonadotrophin (hCG) is given. Regular ultrasound measurements of the developing follicles and checks of blood levels of oestrogen is important. Without this monitoring these drugs can cause dangerous hyperstimulation syndrome (see page 65). Multiple ovulation can also result in multiple birth. By monitoring the response of the ovaries carefully, the triggering dose of hCG can be withheld if there are too many follicles.

Because FSH is expensive, and ultrasound adds to the cost, most clinics offer treatment for only three months at a time. If conception does not follow after six ovulatory cycles, treatment should be stopped as there is a less than 10 per cent chance that continued treatment will be successful. Then IVF is usually indicated.

Pulsatile treatments

In fertile women, the pituitary gland releases FSH and luteinising hormone (LH) in pulses every 60–90 minutes. Doctors have tried to mimic nature by giving pulsatile injections by 'pump therapy'. The patient wears a small electric pump attached to a syringe which delivers precise doses at the most appropriate intervals. Pump therapy has helped women with polycystic ovary disease, and those producing inadequate amounts of FSH and LH.

Releasing hormone
LH and FSH production by the pituitary gland is triggered by the secretion of releasing hormones in the hypothalamus at the base of the brain. Injection of LH-releasing hormone (LHRH) at regular intervals has been an effective treatment in uncommon cases where the communication between the hypothalamus and the pituitary gland is inadequate. LHRH therapy is less likely to cause multiple pregnancy as it merely stimulates the pituitary gland to produce LH and FSH in natural amounts. This treatment can be continued for six months at least before considering IVF.

Wedge resection and ovarian drilling
When drug treatment fails, polycystic ovaries can be treated by removing pieces of ovarian tissue. It is quite unclear why this works; perhaps it alters production of growth factors in the ovary affecting developing follicles. Both laparoscopy or microsurgery make it possible to perform this without the risk of adhesion formation, which can damage the tubes. One common method involves 'drilling' the ovarian capsule with an electric needle or with a laser beam. Incidentally, this may be one reason why some women get pregnant immediately after a failed IVF treatment cycle – egg collection is, after all, somewhat like ovarian drilling.

Other drugs that modify ovulation
There are a number of drugs that modify ovulation, including Buserelin, Lupron and progesterone.

Buserelin and Lupron These drugs are chemically similar LHRH, and initially encourage the pituitary gland to produce more FSH and LH but after several days they suppress it (see page 53). Buserelin is chiefly used with drugs like FSH to stimulate the ovary. In some women, particularly those with polycystic ovaries, it can be more effective to give it initially to suppress pituitary function, then to follow this with FSH so that the ovary becomes highly responsive. This principle is used during IVF treatment, but it can be also used simply to induce ovulation in selected cases. The disadvantage is that it may stimulate the release of too many eggs. It is used more in IVF than for induction of ovulation, as the surplus eggs can be collected, fertilised and stored during an IVF cycle.

The ability of Buserelin to stop ovarian function can be used to suppress hormonally dependent conditions like endometriosis or fibroids, both of which thrive on oestrogen. Once the ovaries are suppressed, endometriosis and fibroids tend to shrink. When Buserelin is stopped this temporary menopause ceases, which can mean the eventual return of endometriosis or regrowth of fibroids.

Progesterone Sometimes, the uterine lining does not develop well; this may occasionally be due to progesterone deficiency. Extra progesterone in the form of an injection or vaginal pessary may help. Alternatively, injections of hCG, which encourage the ovaries to produce progesterone, may have the same effect.

Artificial insemination (AI)

This is the process by which sperm are injected either into the vagina, cervix or more usually the uterus (intrauterine insemination or IUI), at the time of ovulation. It is mostly used when sperm donation is needed. But insemination with a partner's semen, known as 'artificial insemination by husband' (AIH), still has a small place. AI is best done by direct injection into the uterus as this improves the chance of sperm getting into the Fallopian tubes, where fertilisation occurs.

Vaginal or cervical insemination

Semen can be injected into the vagina through a small tube and placed in or near the cervical canal. The woman lies with her knees up for a few minutes, but insemination causes no discomfort. This can be used for couples having difficulties with sex or if the cervix is anatomically abnormal, preventing sperm getting to the right place. This treatment has little point for men with a low sperm count.

Intrauterine insemination

The seminal fluid must be prepared before IUI as unprocessed semen injected into the uterus can cause allergic reactions. The sperm are 'washed' by being repeatedly mixed in special media, then centrifuged to remove debris such as dead cells shed during collection. Sperm can be separated and their numbers enriched. This is done by placing sperm at the bottom of a column of medium. Healthy sperm swim up to the surface and can be collected using a pipette. This is helpful if there are many dead sperm or cells in the semen, or if there are sperm antibodies.

IUI is most effective when the ovaries gently stimulated by either clomiphene or injections of FSH. Stimulation must avoid the risk of multiple follicles being produced. To prevent the risk of twins or more, FSH injections are accompanied by regular ultrasound; it is therefore quite a demanding treatment. Occasionally a split ejaculate (see page 30) will obtain richer sperm.

Although insemination causes little physical discomfort, there may be emotional pain. The process is clinical; unspontaneous and for some, humiliating. The man may find it hard to masturbate to order and the treatment may be embarrassing, occasionally even accompanied by feelings of guilt, frustration and anger. Both partners need patience and understanding. All insemination requires timing of ovulation, but temperature charting is inadequate. To maximise the chances of the sperm being in the right place at the right time, insemination may be repeated two or three times each month. Even so, most couples take several months to conceive. Some find it so disruptive that they give up shortly after starting. If insemination has not worked after six attempts, IVF may be best.

REASONS FOR OFFERING ARTIFICIAL INSEMINATION

AI may be used for a wide variety of reasons:

- When the infertility is unexplained (see page 20).
- If a man has a marginally low sperm count or sperm antibodies. Occasionally, if IVF failed but gave evidence that the sperm were capable of fertilisation, it can just be worth persisting with AI.
- When there are sexual difficulties or possibly inability to have sex at the fertile time. But if this persists, there is a serious chance of frustration or anger, and a risk to the relationship. Every attempt to get psychosexual help is advisable. AI may be justified (with frozen sperm) if the male partner is away from home, but is not ideal, as it may cause considerable stress for the woman.
- If a man has retrograde ejaculation (see page 31).
- When both partners have a minor problem such as irregular ovulation, inability to have regular intercourse, or a slightly marginal sperm count.
- When the woman has upper vaginal or cervical scarring, most commonly after a cone biopsy of the cervix when cancer cells are removed. Artificial insemination by IUI has been successful if the cervix does not produce normal mucus.
- In some cases where the woman does not ovulate regularly, but ovulates in response to drugs like clomiphene or FSH injections. When treatment with these drugs alone has failed, IUI can be added.
- For donor insemination. If there has been no success after several cycles however, IVF with donor sperm may be appropriate, particularly for older women.

Donor insemination

Insemination using sperm from a donor may be appropriate if a man is not producing any viable sperm or if he carries a serious genetic mutation which might be passed to a child. DI is not always successful because the sperm must be frozen during quarantine whilst tests are completed to ensure the donor has no serious illnesses. The freezing/thawing process undoubtedly reduces the fertility of the sperm, and few clinics achieve better than 10–15 per cent chance of a pregnancy per month. Many healthy, perfectly fertile women fail to conceive in spite of multiple attempts at insemination.

In the past, sperm donors in Britain were mostly university students (often studying medicine) because access to them was easy and student doctors often had some limited understanding of what intractable infertility means to a couple; others were married men with children. It has become far harder to recruit donors now that their anonymity is lost. The UK government was under considerable pressure from the offspring of anonymous donation[1] to ensure that a child could always trace its genetic parent when it reached adulthood. Attempts are usually made to match the physical characteristics of the woman's partner, as well as his ethnic group and religion, if requested. The blood group of the donor is matched to avoid risks of the baby developing Rhesus disease.

Less attention is paid to what is as important. University students, often achievers in a particular academic field, may not provide the best match for the background of a recipient, but such considerations are seldom discussed. Sperm donors are not always of proven fertility and may not have had children. They are often unmarried and probably unready for a

---

1   Donor-conceived individuals are now entitled to information about their sperm donor. All donors must register both non-identifying information (such as physical characteristics and medical background) as well as their name and date of birth. This information is provided to the clinic and lodged with the HFEA. Whilst recipients of donor sperm may be given only non-identifying information, those conceived by donor can request non-identifying information at the age of 16 and identifying information from the age of 18. There is little doubt that these rules have greatly reduced the number of men coming forward to offer their reproductive services.

long-term relationship. Nor, of course, can a donor be proved to be free of all genes causing serious inherited disease. Screening for cystic fibrosis is possible but there are around 6,000 other potentially serious genetic conditions. A genetic history of the donor's family does not guarantee freedom from one of these rarer inherited mutations.

If repeated inseminations with a particular donor's semen fail to produce a pregnancy, a different donor may be tried. Donor programmes are likely to have an extremely limited number of fertile donors and inevitably clinics repeatedly use semen from a donor of proved fertility. The fear that siblings conceived by DI might marry, unaware of their relationship to each other, resulted in a ruling that no donor should have his semen used more than ten times[2]. The risk of consanguinity amongst offspring is small, but it exists.

Tubal microsurgery

Regrettably tubal surgery for damaged Fallopian tubes has largely fallen into disuse. In properly selected cases it is unquestionably more successful than IVF. The major advance in tubal surgery was the use of the microscope and very fine instruments. However, microsurgery requires particular skill from the surgeon and too few doctors are now prepared to be trained in it. IVF requires less dexterity and private IVF is such an 'industry' that very few specialists will undertake microsurgery. Worse still, unskilled surgery in the wrong hands or without a microscope is more likely to increase any existing damage by causing adhesions.

Apart from being potentially more successful than IVF, microsurgery treats the underlying cause. Microsurgical repair of the tubes allows patients to become pregnant after natural intercourse, and they often have repeated pregnancies at regular intervals afterwards. There is no increased risk of multiple pregnancy or the other complications associated with IVF. It is sad that more doctors do not consider it, or think of referring patients to a centre where this treatment has good success rates.

---

2   I get the impression that this ruling is not strictly observed because of a national shortage of donors. It is obviously very difficult to enforce.

The main microsurgical procedures

Unless there are good reasons to the contrary, microsurgery should be tried before IVF and it is crucial that the surgeon doing the operation is experienced.

Division or removal of tubal adhesions Adhesions are a very common cause of female infertility. They sometimes occur after infection, or after surgery – for example, an appendicectomy. This operation is called adhesiolysis. It is used to remove adhesions around the ovaries or uterus. Salpingolysis is similar and involves the freeing of the Fallopian tubes. In good hands, and with proper patient selection, the chance of pregnancy is between 40 and 60 per cent.

Opening the ovarian end of the tubes Blockage of the Fallopian tubes near the ovary causes the tube to fill with fluid causing a hydrosalpinx. The operation to open this end of the tube is called salpingostomy. If the hydrosalpinx is large or scarred it is very unlikely to be treatable by surgery; IVF is best. But in suitable patients with less damage, microsurgical salpingostomy can result in one-third of women having a baby.

Unblocking tubes near the uterus The Fallopian tubes can become blocked where they join the uterus in the area called the cornu. Until the advent of microsurgery, the standard (and usually unsuccessful) operation involved removing the cornu and crudely connecting the tube to the uterus. But with a microscope, removal of the blocked or damaged cornu and then stitching the healthy tube together (so-called cornual anastomosis), offers successful pregnancy to between 40 and 55 per cent of women.

Reversal of sterilisation Women who have been sterilised by cutting or tying their tubes can usually have their tubes repaired by microsurgery. The chance of a live birth afterwards is between 65 and 95 per cent, depending mostly on how the sterilisation was done.

Undergoing abdominal tubal microsurgery

The standard procedure involves a cut across the pubic hairline, known a 'bikini' incision, which, after six months, usually leaves a faint scar. Microsurgery can cause such little tissue damage that patients often recover more quickly than after conventional operations. The worst discomfort is usually in the first two days caused by abdominal swelling with wind. Discharge from hospital is usual after three or four days and stitches are removed after seven days. It usually takes at least 6–8 weeks to recover, although some people get back to normal more quickly. There is no harm in having sex as soon as both partners feel up to it[3], but for the first two weeks after leaving hospital it is best not to strain the abdomen by heavy lifting or vigorous exercise. Although the tubes themselves cannot be damaged, overexertion delays healing and causes soreness. The inconvenience associated with microsurgery is no more, and sometimes less, than after IVF.

Regular follow-up is essential every three months until a pregnancy or a decision to try alternative treatments. This enables your surgeon to maximise fertility by keeping an eye, for example, on ovulation. If there are any gynaecological symptoms after surgery, such as pain or irregular bleeding, the specialist should be consulted promptly to check for inflammation or infection. As soon as a woman thinks she is pregnant, she should let her specialist know, as a history of tubal damage increases the chance of ectopic pregnancy. Once there is a positive pregnancy test, monitoring with ultrasound is important.

Women who do not get pregnant immediately after tubal surgery worry about how soon to try IVF. This depends partly on how well the surgeon feels surgery went and the woman's age. Younger women (under 36) might continue trying naturally for at least a year. Some of my patients conceived two or three years after surgery, and after that had repeated pregnancies. We have had one patient who did not conceive for 18 months, then had six live babies at yearly intervals.

Laparoscopic assessment of the Fallopian tubes six months or so after surgery ensures they are open and without adhesions. Women who opt

---

3   One of my patients holds an unconfirmed world record in this respect. In an operating theatre in Texas, I joined her blocked tubes under a microscope on a Wednesday afternoon and on the following Saturday she was caught by a nurse delivering afternoon tea *in flagrante delicto* in bed in a side ward with her boyfriend. The nurse had simply come to ask if she wanted a biscuit. Three weeks later she had a positive pregnancy test – the little girl was subsequently called Mary-Ellen.

for tubal surgery should understand that it is not an instant solution. It is very easy to feel dispirited at the start of a period, especially when it is a day or two late. It is as well to remember that after fertility surgery the chance of conception each month is about 10 per cent, compared to 20 per cent in completely healthy individuals. Most women who had tubal damage of any kind, particularly if there was inflammation, have some ovarian damage. Many of those with extensive damage will have a somewhat reduced chance of a pregnancy. IVF after inflammation is also slightly less likely to be successful.

Laparoscopic surgery

Laparoscopy can avoid open abdominal surgery. The telescope is introduced through a small hole near the navel, and the fine instruments through small holes made just above the pubic hairline. Long scissors, or lasers are used to cut adhesions. Bleeding is controlled using a diathermy machine. This is a particularly useful way of dealing with endometriosis or cysts in the ovaries. One advantage of laparoscopic surgery over abdominal microsurgery is the speed with which patients recover; they generally need to stay in hospital just overnight.

Laparoscopic surgery is most successful when there are adhesions. It is less satisfactory for opening blocked Fallopian tubes. Although the recovery after laparoscopic surgery is rather quicker than with open microsurgery, the pregnancy rate is slightly less.

Tubal catheterisation

Tubal catheterisation is sometimes used for when the tubes are blocked around the cornu. A fine wire probe or dilator can be passed into each tube from below using X-ray monitoring. Optimistic results have been quoted for this procedure, but I am unconvinced. It is only an outpatient procedure but merely dilating the blocked part of the tube will certainly not remove any diseased tissue, so tubal function is still impaired. Some advocates of the operation claim that 40 per cent of their patients conceive.

Treatment for endometriosis

Endometriosis occasionally leads to adhesions or severe scarring of the tubes. Mild or moderate endometriosis only needs treatment when the woman is suffering pain or where there is bad scarring or distortion of the tissues around the tubes and ovaries. Spots of endometriosis can be burned with diathermy. This can also be used for endometriotic cysts in the ovary. Depending on the extent of disease between 30 and 70 per cent of women will conceive after laparoscopic surgery.

Endometriosis is a puzzling disease. It is essentially deposits of the lining of the womb. These can grow (and menstruate) under the influence of oestrogen, so drugs like Buserelin that suppress ovarian activity, also suppress endometriosis (see page 53). Drug therapy reduces the need for surgery, but it can have unpleasant side effects. Also, conception is virtually impossible while these drugs are taken and endometriosis is may regrow after the treatment has been stopped for more than a few months. If the endometriosis is mild, surgery is of no benefit and IVF may best. But whether IVF is really more effective than just having regular sex is open to serious question (see page 19). When the endometriosis is severe, IVF is less successful and surgery has a place. Hormonal stimulation of the ovaries during IVF treatment can stimulate more endometriosis and it is quite common for women with endometriosis to have irregular menstrual cycles or pain after a failed IVF cycle. But any treatment that results in pregnancy encourages suppression of endometriosis; pregnancy hormones inhibit the growth of all endometrial tissue.

Uterine problems

There are many conditions that affect the uterus, causing infertility.

Fibroids

These benign tumours may cause infertility if they distort the uterine cavity, displace the ovaries or block the uterine end (cornu) of the Fallopian tubes. When they distort the anatomy sufficiently to cause infertility, they are best removed microsurgically by myomectomy.

Fibroids can be carefully dissected away from the uterine muscle without causing much disruption of the normal anatomy and the uterus is meticulously repaired with fine stitches. The uterus may bleed and extra blood is usually on hand as a precaution, but transfusion is seldom needed. With a microsurgical approach and specially designed instruments, the risk of any serious blood loss is minimal. Myomectomy is best done by an experienced, qualified fertility expert. When this operation is genuinely indicated in women under the age of 38, about 65 per cent conceive.

Some surgeons use the laparoscope. With laparoscopic instruments or a laser, the fibroids can be shelled out or burnt away. This may cause less post-operative discomfort, but laparoscopic myomectomy can cause more damage, which may prevent the tubes from picking up an egg. Also, the uterine healing can be poor. My impression is that fewer women treated by laparoscopy become pregnant than after open microsurgery.

A third method of myomectomy is embolisation. This blocks the blood supply to the fibroids so that these benign tumours wither. It is usually done under local anaesthesia by a radiologist. A catheter is fed into the artery of one wrist, or into the femoral artery in one leg, under X-ray guidance, then manipulated into the blood vessels supplying the uterus. An embolising agent – usually tiny beads – can be injected to block the fibroid's blood supply, blood flow will shrink or stop completely and the fibroids will die. The procedure, which may be associated with mild pain after it is finished, can take approximately one hour. Although the fibroids can often be dealt with using this method, it is unclear whether it restores fertility as effectively as open surgery. The risks are small, though on very rare occasions infection has occurred. There may also be a risk to the ovaries if the little beads get into the wrong arteries.

Congenital abnormalities of the womb
During early development, the uterus grows from two separate tubes, which fuse during intrauterine life. Most congenital abnormalities result from incomplete fusion and can cause infertility or miscarriage. Rarely,

an abdominal operation to correct this defect is advisable and around 65 per cent of women will conceive. Most abnormalities are not that severe and can be tackled through the vagina by day-case surgery. Most common is a septate uterus, when the upper part of the uterine cavity is deformed by a bridge of tissue – a division or septum. This can usually be cut away using a telescope – a hysteroscope – passed from the vagina. There may be some vaginal bleeding afterwards, usually less than a period. The surgeon may place a coil in the uterus afterwards to keep the walls of the uterus separate for 2–4 weeks. The chance of pregnancy is about 75 per cent.

IVF should not be tried until attempts are made to correct any uterine abnormality. A common cause for IVF failure is an undiagnosed congenital deformity of the uterus. These defects are often missed because a hysterosalpingogram X-ray (see HSG, page 40) of the uterus is not done first. I feel like weeping when I see women who **have** had four or five failed IVF attempts, finding that a simple day-case procedure to correct uterine problems was all that was needed.

Internal adhesions of the womb

Internal adhesions known as synechiae or Asherman's syndrome, often cause the wall of the uterine cavity to stick together and are best diagnosed by HSG. They can usually be separated with a hysteroscope (see page 43) using fine scissors or a laser and the operation can be done as a day-case. Surgery may need to be repeated, sometimes more than once, and it may be necessary to insert a plastic coil into the uterus for a few weeks to keep the uterine walls apart during healing. The chance of pregnancy afterwards depends on the extent of the adhesions. IVF is never indicated until every reasonable attempt at correcting adhesions has been made.

Polyps

These are fleshy, grape-like growths on the wall of the inside of the uterus. They can be removed by a D&C (dilation of the cervix and curettage), or 'scrape', on the rare occasions when they are a cause of infertility.

Adenomyosis

The uterus can become scarred when its muscle is invaded by lining tissue (the endometrium). Surgery is usually not effective as the tissue cannot normally be removed without uterine damage. Like endometriosis, drugs that suppress ovarian activity will cause the tissue to shrink, but also prevent ovulation during their use. One alternative treatment is embolisation, using the same approach as used for fibroids (see page 130). Women with adenomyosis have at most only a 35 per cent chance of getting pregnant. Sadly IVF has a poor chance of success; depending on its severity success rates seem to vary from 5–15 per cent.

Mixing sperm and egg

Before IVF had been developed, the late Professor McClure Browne experimented at Hammersmith Hospital with mixing egg and sperm together and inserting them into the Fallopian tubes. So in the 1960s, when an infertile patient was scheduled for exploratory surgery[4], he might ask his trainee assistants to prepare some infertile patients by stimulating ovulation using clomiphene. Surgery would be scheduled for just before ovulation was expected. The husband's sperm was collected and I well remember many lengthy and painstaking attempts to use my trembling fingers to direct a fine piece of plastic tubing containing the sperm into the Fallopian tubes under his unforgiving gaze. The subsequent invention of the laparoscope did not greatly simplify matters, as trying to insert the tubing through a tiny hole in the abdomen was rather like one of those fairground devices where you guide a model crane behind a glass panel to pick up a present. As far as I know, Professor McClure Brown pioneered this approach and sometimes he would try to suck an egg from the follicle in the ovary at the same time – years before gamete intra-Fallopian transfer (GIFT)

---

4   It seems amazing now, but when I was in training there was very little we could do for infertile women and it was quite usual to do a laparotomy (open the abdomen under anaesthesia) to see if there was a problem that could be corrected surgically. When laparoscopy became available there were fewer unnecessary major operations.

was invented in California. He never published this work, but there were occasional pregnancies. I mention tubal insemination through pure nostalgia.

Gamete intra-Fallopian transfer

Known as GIFT, this is now largely obsolescent, but has a place for patients who have religious objections to creating a human embryo in culture. It involves stimulation of the ovaries to produce eggs, collecting them from the ovaries, then mixing them with sperm. Immediately after mixing (and before fertilisation) both are placed in the Fallopian tube of the woman. The treatment differs from IVF because the eggs are not fertilised; fertilisation occurs in its natural environment, the Fallopian tube. This may seem an advantage, but the results are generally worse than with IVF.

The treatment, unlike IVF, does not bypass the Fallopian tube and consequently is not appropriate where there is tubal disease. GIFT is most effective when more than one egg has been collected and mixed with the sperm. Therefore, as with IVF, there is a risk of overstimulation of the ovaries. It also needs an operation to collect the eggs, which are usually collected by laparoscopy (see page 42), rather than ultrasound, because the surgeon generally uses the laparoscope to put the eggs and sperm into the Fallopian tube.

GIFT was usually used for unexplained infertility. As it bypasses the cervix, it has also been used when there is a problem with the cervical mucus, but it is not as effective as IVF. It is obviously better to transfer embryos knowing that fertilisation and embryo development are normal, rather than returning unfertilised eggs that may or may not develop. GIFT attempts are limited, too, because IVF gives better information. As access to IVF has greatly improved, GIFT has become less fashionable. But because the procedure does not produce an embryo inside the body, it can be done in any hospital and is not licensed by law. Oddly, the HFEA has no control over it. Whilst it may be more acceptable for some patients such as religious Catholics, because embryos are not produced in vitro, it is still procreation without sexual intercourse.

Zygote intra-Fallopian transfer

Known as ZIFT, this is a variation on GIFT treatment, but involves placing a fertilised egg (zygote) in the Fallopian tube. In ZIFT, eggs are collected as for IVF, fertilised outside the body in vitro, and when fertilised, one or two are selected for transfer into the Fallopian tube, normally using laparoscopy. The thinking behind the technique is that by placing the very early fertilised egg into the Fallopian tube, it will be in its most natural environment. In practice, however, there seems a small advantage. It is as complicated as IVF, and like GIFT requires laparoscopy. Moreover, if there is any damage to the Fallopian tube there may be a risk of ectopic pregnancy.

Chapter 10: Taking control of your treatment

During a such a complex and emotionally charged process as IVF it is common to feel out of control. There are a number of things you can do to help you feel in charge. Where you start, and how you proceed from there, are positive choices you can make.

Your general practitioner (GP)

The point of departure for most couples seeking fertility treatment is their family doctor. Unfortunately many doctors (and even some consultant gynaecologists) have too little knowledge of the clinics they recommend. Their experience of IVF is sometimes minimal, and couples are sometimes more likely to get reliable information through their own efforts. But a good GP is the best person to give you general advice and can have an important role throughout diagnosis and treatment.

To find the criteria for NHS funding and treatment in your area, you should talk to your GP. Failing that, your local NHS Health Commissioning Group may be able to advise. Bear in mind that there will be waiting lists for NHS treatment, which vary according to the particular authority. Waiting lists are not generally the fault of the IVF clinic – at present this is entirely dependent on the degree of funding that the local health commissioner has agreed to provide.

You are entitled to seek treatment as a private patient and an NHS patient at the same time, but you will need separate referral letters from your GP. Some Health Authorities may withhold NHS treatment from patients who have already had private treatment. This is something that you may need to check locally.

Choosing a clinic

IVF in the UK has a very high standard. Most clinics are honest, caring and competent. There have been remarkable improvements in reproductive medicine over the last few years. There is a training programme, and there are more excellent doctors practising than ever before. The Human Fertilisation and Embryology Authority (HFEA) has also played its part. Whatever the limitations of regulation, the HFEA has consistently tried to improve the information given to patients and the standard of treatment and counselling they receive. Now the NHS has to understand that, for too long, it has not regarded these treatments as being sufficiently important.

There are several organisations concerned with infertility that can provide information. The HFEA publishes a guide: 'Getting started – your guide to fertility treatment', which can be downloaded from its website. The website claims 'If you're exploring fertility treatment, the HFEA is the first place to go for reliable information. Our expertise and years of experience mean we can provide you with authoritative, independent information'. Regrettably, there is much information missing from the website. It has virtually nothing on the reason for trying to make a diagnosis before starting IVF, has little to offer you if IVF fails (which of course happens in two-thirds of cycles) and also, it stresses relatively unimportant aspects of 'lifestyle', but almost totally ignores the serious issue of weight, which remains one of the most common reasons for failure of treatment, complications after it and during pregnancy. The leading self-help group is Infertility Network UK IVF, but unfortunately nearly all the groups that give advice do seem on occasion to be fairly limited or funded by manufacturers that may have vested interests. The Genesis Research Trust tries hard to avoid bias while providing independent expertise.

What to consider

If you are lucky enough to a) have funding, and b) have a choice of clinic, you may wish to consider the following issues, which are relevant to those considering NHS or private treatment.

- Did you like and feel confident with the clinic's doctors and nurses? Did they seem like a team? If so, good communication, so vital to the treatment, is likely to be adequate.
- Do patients regularly see a doctor rather than a member of the paramedical staff? Can you see the same person during treatment? Good units try to ensure continuity of care and communication.
- Does the clinic do adequate tests to establish a clear diagnosis before treatment? This may seem beyond the competence of a lay person to decide, but it is fairly simple to find out, for example, if the doctors take a uterine X-ray or hysterosalpingogram (see HSG, page 40) or personally examine X-rays taken earlier or at another hospital. If you merely ask, 'Do you do the necessary tests?' clinic staff may simply say 'Yes'. So you could ask, for example, specific questions about the tests that the clinic finds are important in unexplained infertility.
- Does the clinic also do key tests, such as hormone tests, at the beginning of the menstrual cycle, detailed scans, proper sperm function tests, before committing a patient to IVF? Beware of the specialist who only offers you the expensive lucrative tests – such as laparoscopy – especially if they offer them first.
- Does the clinic have an independent counsellor offering a free service? Couples should have the opportunity to talk to someone who has not been involved in their treatment and can offer them objective advice. This person should not be involved in giving clinical information, but rather in helping you to feel comfortable about what is happening.
- Does the clinic provide a comprehensive range of fertility treatments? Be wary of clinics that offer IVF as their main or only treatment, or offer it to the exclusion of other techniques. This is convenient for them, but may not be in the best interests of their patients.
- How thoroughly is each treatment cycle monitored? Generally, clinics

that do regular hormone tests, for example, get better results and may have fewer complications. They will also have a better idea of what went wrong if the treatment fails.

- Does the clinic have a fixed drugs regime for stimulating women to produce eggs, or do they tailor it the treatment to suit individuals and their circumstances?
- Are careful and repeated assessments of sperm quality made before IVF treatment is begun? A good unit will have a set of precisely worked-out values for sperm quality, and will cancel an attempt if it thinks that there is no chance of fertilisation.
- Is it possible to make weekend appointments if you have a problem? Does the clinic offer egg collections and inseminations most days of the week? If they can only do treatments two or three times a week, your success may be jeopardised.
- Is there a choice of local or general anaesthesia and is an anaesthetist present during egg collection to ensure safety?
- How many embryos does the clinic routinely put back into the uterus? Clinics putting more than one embryo back in women under 35, are often taking risks to improve pregnancy rates.
- How much does the clinic charge? If it charges much more than other clinics, they may be overcharging. Costs should be inclusive apart from drugs. Be wary of any clinic that charges huge hidden costs, for example, for extra ultrasound examinations, additional consultations, and pregnancy tests.
- If the treatment fails, will you see the director of the clinic personally? The director or somebody who holds the equivalent of an NHS consultant post should be available (by appointment) to see couples whose treatment cycle fails. He or she should discuss the progress of the cycle, working out what, if anything, went wrong, where improvements are needed, and to advise on whether a further IVF attempt or other treatment should be considered.

Assessing a clinic's published results

The first thing to understand is that comparison of results between clinics is almost meaningless. Even if one clinic reports a success rate of say 27 per cent, and another only 10 per cent, there may be no statistical difference. Unless the clinics are publishing results from a very large number of patients – say over 500–1,000 a year – careful analysis by competent statisticians shows comparisons are meaningless. The results in any clinic depend primarily on the kind of patient they are treating: their age, their cause of infertility, the length they have been trying to conceive, the number of cycles of IVF (with or without ICSI) that a couple has failed, and the response of their ovaries to drugs.

These factors vary hugely between clinics. Remember too, that data collection and publication take a long time and any reported figures are, on average, over two years old.

Some clinics have quite high cancellation rates before egg collection if they feel there is a poor chance of success. In most cases, this will be an attempt to save their patients money, because cycles stopped before egg collection are generally charged at a fraction of the total cost. However, a high cancellation rate may result in published success rates looking rather better than those of another clinic that does not cancel so early.

Clinics with more than around 600 cycles annually are larger and tend to be more successful. A clinic should also have enough data to be able to provide a computerised breakdown of your chance of success in your particular circumstance based on results from similar patients.

Some thoughts about the treatment of unexplained Infertility

I feel I need to write something here that may be as unpopular with many of my colleagues, as it will be disturbing for many patients who opt for IVF or intrauterine insemination. In recent years a great deal of research has gone into the medical management of unexplained infertility and it is clear, from various studies, that in many centres around the world, there is much overtreatment. That is to say that many of the regular methods of helping people with unexplained infertility are quite unnecessary.

Over 20 years ago two colleagues, Patrick Taylor and John Collins, wrote a detailed account of the subject in their book, *Unexplained*

Infertility, now sadly out of print[1]. In a book of over 250 pages, they wrote what I consider to be the best account of unexplained infertility ever written. Whilst showing huge sympathy and great sensitivity towards couples with this 'diagnosis', they gave a detailed mathematical analysis. They evaluated the likelihood of getting pregnant when, after careful diagnosis, this condition was treated by various means, including IVF. What they showed was that most of the treatments that had been used had not been properly compared with no treatment at all. In essence, what their book reports is that virtually all treatments that are used are no better than doing nothing. I can do no better than to quote the last paragraph of their penultimate chapter:

'… on the issue of efficacy, however, only clomiphene therapy has been demonstrated by means of acceptable clinical evidence in the form of randomised trials as a treatment with proven superiority of no therapy. On the basis of best available evidence, hMG (gonadotrophins) plus intrauterine insemination has possible but unproven benefit, and no studies exist to demonstrate a benefit for in vitro fertilisation methodology'.

Over 20 years later, their position certainly seems to be still justified. In January 2015, Dr Fleur Kersten from Nijmegen, Holland, and her colleagues, published an important study on this subject[2]. They collected records from 25 clinics and identified 544 infertile couples who had been carefully examined and who had no clearly identifiable cause for their infertility. The average length they had been infertile was 18 months. The patients they define as having unexplained infertility included a number of women who only had one tube clearly open, some had mild male infertility (motile sperm count ranging from 3–10 million) and some mild endometriosis (they excluded any female patient over the age of 38).

Of the identified couples, 198 had had what Dr Kersten called overtreatment – that is, within six months of presenting with infertility

---

1   *Unexplained Infertility*, Patrick J. Taylor and John A. Collins, Oxford University Press, New York and Oxford, 1992.

2   'Overtreatment in couples with unexplained infertility', F.A.M. Kersten *et al*, *Human Reproduction* 2015, Jan;30(1):71–80.

they had been given ovarian stimulation or IVF. The remaining 346 couples had no treatment, but were simply followed expectantly for one year. In the treated group, 28 per cent became pregnant within six months of starting the survey, and in the untreated group 31 per cent had a pregnancy. After one year, 42 per cent in the treated group became pregnant and 41 per cent in the untreated group. Eventually, 90 per cent of the treated group had a pregnancy, compared with 91 per cent in the untreated group who had a pregnancy naturally.

I find this study not only interesting but also, in a curious way, extremely reassuring. First, the authors point out that treatment often seemed to delay the much-wanted successful outcome. Secondly, some mild causes of infertility, for example, an apparently rather low sperm count, does not condemn anxious couples to a life of sterility. Thirdly, it is very clear that after thorough testing and a diagnosis of genuinely unexplained infertility, there is an excellent chance of having a pregnancy naturally without expensive treatment. Perhaps the message should be 'Just think of the number of women who have got pregnant spontaneously after several treatment cycles have failed.'

So should you try IVF again?

Probably the most important job that I did when in charge of a large clinic was to see personally as many patients as I could who had failed an IVF cycle. The couples who came after failure nearly always asked one question, 'Should we try again?' This is possibly the most complicated question in the whole of reproductive medicine and good advice is difficult. Firstly, it is clear that the cause of the infertility, properly investigated, is particularly important.

Remember that, in any case, failure is merely statistically probable. Please do understand that, overall, each IVF cycle only has around a one in four chance of success because even in nature most human embryos do not implant. If you placed your money on a horse at four to one against and it had not won, you would not think that there was anything surprising about this result. Much of the time, going through a repeated cycle is merely improving natural odds.

There are assessments you need to make. You cannot always expect the doctor at your clinic to tell what you should do because good doctors feel it quite presumptuous to tell patients to continue or to stop. Here are some questions that may be helpful in trying to assess to this most difficult decision.

How did you both feel about the treatment?

For some people, going through IVF is a harrowing experience, one that they do not wish to repeat. For others, it is much easier than expected and they find that there is much that is positive. I have no doubt, therefore, that one of the questions that should be top of this list, is your own assessment of how you found the treatment. If you found it depressing or difficult, you should think seriously before trying again; I would strongly advise talking to a third person.

Good clinics offer in-house counselling with a professional who has great expertise in helping people to pinpoint what their feelings really are. Far too often, people underestimate the value of good counselling. No counsellor will be able to tell you what to do, but he or she will help you focus on the crucial aspects of how you feel, to make your own mature judgement about further treatment.

Can we afford it?

This is a question not asked enough. IVF is expensive and subsequent treatment cycles may cost even more. As a woman gets older, she may need more follicle stimulating hormone (FSH) to stimulate the ovaries. It is not uncommon for the amount to increase with successive treatment cycles, and for costs to spiral. You may need to be serious about whether it might be better to spend your money in other ways. This, I think, is particularly true for those who already have one child. Sometimes it may be better to consider spending the money on your existing family, rather than forlornly trying to increase it.

Regrettably, the regulatory authority, the HFEA has done far too little to change what is charged both in the private sector, and also in the NHS. But it is ludicrous that an NHS cycle of treatment may cost £1,000 in some parts of the country and the same treatment in others over £5,000. And in private clinics it is common for a couple to have paid far more than this by the time a single IVF treatment is concluded. And it is ridiculous, for example, that one clinic may charge £400 for freezing embryos for one year, when a pint of liquid nitrogen in which the embryos are stored costs merely a few pence. It is not as though embryos, invisible to the naked eye, occupy hugely expensive space.

The HFEA has repeatedly claimed it has no power to control fees but this is nonsense. It has the remit to ensure ethical treatment and ethical research, and it has the most significant power of all, to remove a clinic's licence to practise. Infertile patients are vulnerable and easily exploited. It surely is up to the government's own regulatory body to protect them at least as well as any purchaser of other services and commodities who would normally be far better protected.

What does the computer indicate?
More larger clinics now have data of a large number of treatment cycles. These databases can analyse over 600 cycles a year. Some clinics have existed for a long time with broad experience of the various medical conditions impinging on the chances of success. All good clinics keep computer records and most can assess the mathematical chances of failure given another treatment cycle in your situation. It is reasonable to ask, for example, 'Given a patient of my age, with tubal disease, one previous pregnancy, and two failed attempts at IVF, what are the chances if I undertake a third cycle?' Clearly to answer this kind of question accurately from the computer a unit needs a very large database – there are four variables in it – age, tubal damage, previous pregnancy, and considering a third cycle attempt. But those that have records from several thousand patients may be able to provide some insight into your difficult decision. The computer cannot answer everything. For some people, a 3 per cent chance is worth taking; for others, a 15 per cent chance is not.

Are there genetic factors affecting your failure?
Some women have a family history of an earlier than average menopause. It is worth finding out how old your mother was when you were born and how old she was at the birth of your brothers or

sisters. The age when your mother stopped having periods may also help. Women whose mothers tended to have an early menopause may, in turn, have an earlier than average menopause. Under these circumstances it could be worth trying treatment sooner, particularly if there has been a poor response to ovarian stimulation. Assessment of FSH and anti-mullerian hormone (AMH), the number of follicles seen and the volume of the ovaries on ultrasound, will help these decisions.

Have your previous treatment cycles been assessed?
This is important. A visit to the clinic for a troubleshooting session after failed IVF needs perusal of your medical and laboratory records. There are a number of pointers that will suggest whether or not a further treatment may have a good prognosis.

Response to stimulation Patients who require only a small amount of gonadotrophin may have a much better chance should they repeat IVF. This also tends to be true of patients with a tendency to hyperstimulation. Conversely, those women who need massive doses of drugs to induce ovulation are likely to have a poorer prognosis.

Egg numbers Women yielding a reasonable number of eggs, say more than seven or eight, have statistically better chances in another cycle, than those that have produced five or fewer. The number of eggs collected after stimulation is partly dependent on age. Most clinics will be able to tell you the average numbers of eggs they would expect. If you produced rather fewer than the average for your age, it is an indication that another treatment cycle is less likely to be successful.

If you have had several treatment cycles, then adding up the total number of eggs you have produced may also be helpful. Moreover, if the number of eggs is decreasing with each attempt, this suggests reduced chances.

Oestrogen levels Many units take blood samples to measure oestrogen during the treatment cycle. These are a useful indication of how well the ovary has responded and what is the chance of a repeated response. Some units pay attention to the peak oestrogen value, the highest level achieved, usually just before the egg collection. Women with low oestrogen levels, say below 2,500pmols per litre, may have a poorer chance of success in further cycles. As successive cycles are undertaken, the ovaries may become increasingly refractive, that is they tend to fail to respond. Poor response in general carries a poor prognosis in future. Like egg numbers, this may be age related. Nevertheless, a woman of 42 or 43 who produces peak oestrogen levels of more than 5,000pmols per litre may have a better chance.

Fertilisation rate Women who produce poor-quality eggs tend to have a low fertilisation rate. The average, not using ICSI, should be around 60 per cent. Patients who are falling well below that with normal sperm may produce eggs that do not give viable embryos. Poor fertilisation rates, seen repeatedly over several cycles, are not good news. Some clinics try to get round this problem by forcing fertilisation with ICSI. I think it is questionable whether ICSI is really of much benefit in such circumstances. One cannot force a bad egg to become a good embryo simply by injecting a sperm.

Spare embryos A previous treatment cycle may have generated a number of spare embryos, which have been frozen. Sometimes they will have been grown for a while in culture. Observations made on the culture can be valuable. If a number of these embryos grew to the blastocyst stage, this is pretty good evidence that you are producing better-than-average embryos. Clinics often tell patients that their embryos 'look good down the microscope'. As said earlier, it is impossible to tell whether an embryo is good or bad, merely by looking at it (see page 58). But some units do research on spare embryos, and it is your prerogative to have access to these results. The research embryologist's observations on these embryos may give some real clues as to how good the embryos that you produce are.

Preimplantation genetic and biochemical screening (PGS) It is now possible to do molecular tests on embryos. The results tell us more about the chromosomes within the embryos as well as the chemicals they are producing. In future, these tests may be increasingly valuable when used on spare embryos that were not transferred. By examining spare embryos future tests may give a helpful clues to the viability of the embryos from the same batch that were transferred.

USING DONOR EGGS

Women who have a poor response to ovarian stimulation, or who produce very poor eggs that do not fertilise well, may be better treated with an egg from a donor (see page 101). This major decision should certainly be preceded by thorough counselling. It is worth emphasising that there are far more women seeking a donor egg than there are women prepared to give up their eggs. One hopes that in the future, with improvements in technology, donor eggs may become more available. In my view, you should not attempt using donor eggs if there is any reasonable chance that you can produce your own. It is my impression that some clinics tend to offer donor treatment too early, before all else has been explored.

Failed pregnancy If a previous IVF cycle has ended with a failed pregnancy the chance of successful pregnancy in another cycle may be better than average. This is true whether the pregnancy was an ectopic, a miscarriage, or merely an early biochemical pregnancy. Women who have had a child in the last four or five years also seem to have better chances and it may be worthwhile persisting with further IVF attempts. This seems to be true whether the pregnancy was conceived spontaneously or by IVF.

Before another IVF cycle

There a number of tests that need to be carried out before a decision is made to start another cycle of IVF, but there are also some things you can do to help your chances.

FSH and AMH

FSH secretion tends to rise as the ovaries fail. FSH should be measured between days 5 and 9 of an unstimulated cycle before deciding on a repeat IVF attempt. AMH is equally useful. Unfortunately the results of this test are not fully standardised so care is needed in interpretation (see page 38). If the FSH level is much over 10 international units, then the chance of further IVF being successful is reduced and if it is above 15 international units, they are very poor indeed. It is virtually never worth considering IVF if the level is over 20 international units. Once the FSH level has been found to be raised – even if the level returns to normal values – the prognosis is still bad.

Ultrasound assessment

Ovarian ultrasound allows assessment of the total volume of each ovary, giving some indication of ovarian reserve. Patients with very small ovaries, say below a volume of 3mm, are likely to respond less well.

Checking the uterus

An assessment of the uterus should be done before any fertility treatments. If it has not been done (or not within the last three or four years) accurate information about the uterine cavity and its surrounding muscle is useful. Although units frequently offer a hysteroscopy, a better test is undoubtedly HSG. It is cheaper, and done properly with good techniques, not painful. It gives valuable information about the condition of the uterine cavity and whether there are recent changes. There may be defects in the cavity that can be corrected before another IVF attempt, or fibroids that should be removed.

Chromosome assessment

Some men and women have unexpected, undiagnosed chromosome problems giving rise to infertility. It may be worth getting blood tests from both partners if the cause of failure remains puzzling. These tests are not cheap. Ideally, a large number of blood white cells should be examined and not just the routine one or two. This is because some people are 'mosaic'. That is to say, they have some cells that have a normal chromosome complement and others that do not (see page 95). Even 'mosaic' patients may have a higher risk of producing abnormal embryos and a chance of infertility or miscarriage.

What you must do

A commitment to your health, weight and fitness are all regarded as ways you can increase your chances of success when undertaking fertility treatment.

Body weight Even mild obesity (or worse) is a very significant reason for all assisted conception treatments to fail. I most strongly advise you, if you are contemplating any fertility treatment, to try to get to as close to a normal weight as possible. Merely being a few points above normal BMI can halve your chance of success. If you are still overweight and have failed an IVF treatment cycle, it really is silly not to do everything to get to a normal weight. This will almost certainly mean diet, but also regular exercise. It is unwise to go through IVF treatment starving so best to wait until your body weight is in equilibrium. Similarly, women who are underweight also risk failure, have a higher chance of miscarriage and more serious complications during pregnancy – if they conceive at all.

General fitness There is not much evidence one way or another as to whether general fitness makes much difference. However, there is some evidence that smoking, and very excessive alcohol consumption might reduce the chances of getting normal eggs. These excesses certainly reduce the chances of producing normal sperm. While the evidence is poor that these factors make much different to the eggs, it does not make sense to attempt treatments in a toxic state. I do not believe that there is serious evidence that mild alcohol use is detrimental, in spite of the advice on the HFEA's website. Similarly the evidence that coffee is harmful is very poor.

Alternative treatments

There are a number of other alternative treatments that can be explored before embarking on further cycles of IVF.

Short protocol

As women get older, they respond less well to gonadotrophins. If you had a poor response to stimulation last time and are in the older age group, it might be worth discussing short protocol with your doctor (see page 136). With these treatments, Buserelin or similar drugs are only given for a very short time, and gonadotrophins started before FSH is suppressed. Some units have had a better success rate with this in older women, or in those with a poor response to stimulation.

Water on a Fallopian tube (hydrosalpinx)

It is clear from various statistics that if you have tubal disease your chances are less good. There is loose evidence that patients with blocked Fallopian tubes containing fluid do less well than those with normal tubes, or damaged tubes not containing fluid. Some doctors recommend removing blocked, swollen tubes by laparoscopy before IVF. Alternatively, they apply a clip across the tube where it joins the uterus. This is thought to prevent infected fluid inside the Fallopian tube draining into the uterine cavity, so reducing the chance of it altering the uterine environment. There is no statistically proven evidence that such treatments increase the results of IVF.

Treatment of tubal disease

Many women have tubal damage and repeated IVF has failed, but they have not had an operation on their Fallopian tubes. In suitable cases, providing the patients are carefully investigated and selected, the results of tubal surgery are better than IVF. This is particularly the case if the tubal surgery is done with proper microsurgery and an experienced surgeon (see page 126). At Hammersmith Hospital, 42 patients who between them had failed no fewer than 95 treatment cycles of IVF, had 21 live births after tubal surgery for completely blocked tubes. Two of them had already had five IVF attempts each. Even better results were obtained after division of adhesions or removal of fibroids.

Some women just do not respond well to ovarian stimulation. These women may do better with tubal surgery. It is interesting that some patients we have treated successfully with tubal microsurgery, were very poor responders to the drugs to stimulate ovulation.

When should we give up treatment?

It is not sensible to continue IVF against all odds. Many women feel that they wish to gamble, but they may be betting with their health and with their well-being. If you have been through IVF more than twice, and have had consistent testing, then you can know that you have left no reasonable stone unturned. This is an important consideration. You should not have endless repeated treatments, unless the portents clearly indicate some reasonable chance of success, and you have not found earlier treatments too demanding.

Whilst you are a patient, your situation remains unresolved. Do not end up 'enjoying' being a patient – that is getting psychological support from treatment and avoiding the inevitable. All of us, at sometime in our lives, have to lose something we most value. When we lose a parent, for example, we have to mourn, but we do get over this terrible blow. Giving up infertility treatment is not unlike this. Taking the decision to stop, deciding to go through a period of mourning, can be a positive experience. You may feel desperate at the time, but will come out of it much stronger. Once you have made the decision to stop, your whole life can be resolved and you can get on with other valuable things within it.

During the course of this handbook, I have written many things that are depressing. What I have not said much about is that infertility treatment can be an enriching experience. This may sound strange, but so many couples find that it has strengthened their relationship and enabled them to deal with other problems in a more sensible and focused way. Infertile people can allow their treatment to destroy the relationships they most value. It is unwise to let this happen to you. It is worth recognising that you have gone through definitive treatment and may now need to close the door.

Glossary

Adenomyosis When the lining of the womb – the endometrium – grows deep into the muscular wall of the uterus.

Adhesion After infection or trauma, organs often become stuck together with scar tissue. Adhesions are a common cause of female infertility as they may interfere with tubal or ovarian function.

Amino acids The building blocks from which proteins are made.

Asherman's syndrome Where severe adhesions form inside the uterine cavity, sometimes even obliterating it.

Azoospermia When no sperm are produced in the semen.

Biopsy Removal of a small piece of tissue for diagnostic examination under a microscope.

Blastocyst The cluster of cells that develops from a fertilised egg around five days after fertilisation; by this time it will have as many as 160 cells.

Chromosome Tiny string-like structures in the nucleus of each cell in the body containing genes. Humans have 23 paired chromosomes, one half of each pair from the mother, the other from the father.

Corpus luteum After ovulation, the follicle which released the egg becomes a corpus luteum or 'yellow body'. It produces progesterone.

Cryopreservation Preserving tissue, embryos, sperm or eggs by freezing. The process requires various precautions to prevent damage caused by ice crystals.

Cyst A pocket of tissue usually filled with fluid, that can develop anywhere but commonly on the ovary, or testis. Most cysts are not cancerous.

Depot injection Long-acting subcutaneous or intramuscular injection.

Down's syndrome A chromosomal disorder in which there are three copies of chromosome 21 rather than two.

DNA Short for deoxyribonucleic acid, the self-replicating material present in living organisms. DNA, in the form of genes, is packed on chromosomes and contains your genetic information.

Embryo The early stages of growth of a baby, from fertilisation to the beginning of the third month of pregnancy, after which is it called a foetus.

Endometriosis When the endometrium grows into other structures in the abdomen, such as the ovaries, bowel or peritoneum, leading to adhesions or scarring. It is often very mild and may not cause infertility.

Ectopic pregnancy A pregnancy implanting outside the uterus – for example in the Fallopian tube or ovary. It may cause internal bleeding and generally needs prompt treatment.

Epididymis Fine, coiled tube that carries sperm from a testis to the vas deferens.

Fetus Stage of prenatal development of a baby from 12 weeks to birth.

Follicle The cyst-like structure in which each egg develops in the ovary. Just before ovulation, a follicle is around 2cm (½in) in diameter.

Follicle stimulating hormone (FSH) The hormone released by the pituitary gland that stimulates follicles to grow in women and the production of sperm in men. FSH works in conjunction with LH.

Genetic disorder Caused by abnormalities in a person's genes and may be passed onto any offspring.

Gonadotrophins Hormones produced by the pituitary gland which stimulate the ovaries or testes. They can be given by injection during fertility treatment.

HFEA (Human Fertilisation and Embryology Authority) The body set up by government in 1990 which had the remit to regulate good ethical practice in infertility treatments.

Human chorionic gonadotropin (hCG) The hormone produced during pregnancy by the cells that will form the placenta.

Hypothalamus A region at the base of the brain which controls much of the activity of the pituitary gland.

Hysterosalpingogram (HSG) An X-ray of the womb and tubes after injection of a dye. Done carefully, it is the best test to assess the inside of the uterus and condition of the tubes.

Hysteroscopy Telescope inspection of the inside of the womb which may help diagnose polyps, fibroids or adhesions.

Karotype Identification of a person's chromosomes under a powerful microscope.

Laparoscopy A telescope is passed through a small hole near the navel under general anaesthetic. The most informative test in female infertility, providing excellent views and photographs of the tubes, uterus and ovaries.

Luteinising hormone (LH) Hormone released by the pituitary gland that triggers ovulation, or sperm development in men.

Morula An early stage of embryo development, around three days or so after fertilisation.

Mutagen An agent, such as a chemical, that causes genetic mutation. Excessive tobacco and sunlight can be mutagens.

NICE (National Institute for Health and Care Excellence) Government body with the remit to test efficacy of medical treatments.

Oestrogen The main female hormone produced by the cells inside a follicle.

Progesterone Hormone produced by the ovary during the second half of the cycle, after ovulation.

Peritoneum The lining or fine membrane which covers all organs inside the abdomen except the ovaries.

Pituitary agonist drugs Drugs that first stimulate the pituitary gland and then prevent it producing further FSH.

Pituitary gland The 'master gland' which controls most hormonal function. It is attached to the hypothalamus under the brain.

Polycystic ovaries Ovaries may produce multiple cystic follicles without ovulating. When this causes infertility it is referred to

as 'polycystic ovary syndrome' or PCOS.

Polycystic ovary syndrome (PCOS) A common cause of infertility and may be associated with excessive weight, extra growth of hair, irregular periods and failure to ovulate. It can usually be treated with drugs without needing IVF.

Polyp Small growth, usually with a stalk, that projects from cells lining the uterus or tubes. They are nearly always benign but may justify removal if they are distorting the interior of the uterus.

Preimplantation genetic diagnosis Removal of embryonic cells to analyse the DNA to identify genetic disease.

Preimplantation genetic screening Removal of embryonic cells with the hope of determining whether a particular embryo is likely to develop into a baby.

Reactive oxygen species (ROS) Chemically reactive molecules containing oxygen. When raised (for example after stress) they can interfere with the normal working of cells and tissues

Reduced ovarian reserve As women get older, the number of eggs and follicles falls. When only a few eggs are left, this is referred to as reduced ovarian reserve. May cause infertility in younger women.

Spermatogenesis The process of making new sperm cells in the tubules inside the testis.

Testosterone The main male hormone promoting development of male characteristics. It is also produced by cells in the follicle and important for ovulation .

Ultrasound scan High-frequency sound waves can be passed through the body painlessly and the reflected echoes can build up an image of an organ on a computer screen.

Vas deferens Also called the ductus deferens (carrying away vessel), this is the tube that carries the sperm from the epididymis towards the penis.

Zona (or Zona pellucida) The outer covering or 'shell' of an egg.

Zygote The cell formed by the union of two gametes (egg and sperm) before cell division (cleavage) begins.

Index

Dedication

To the many well-trained and altruistic doctors entering the most rewarding career of reproductive medicine. They will recognise the vulnerability of infertile couples and also the foundation of all good medical treatment. Wherever possible to make serious attempts at establishing an accurate diagnosis before offering therapy that is based on sound scientific evidence.

Genesis Research Trust

www.genesisresearchtrust.com

Despite countless breakthroughs in medical science, we still do not understand why some pregnancies will end in tragedy. For most of us, having a child of our own is the most fulfilling experience of our lives. All of us can imagine the desperation and sadness of parents who lose a baby, and the life-shattering impact that a disabled or seriously ill child has on a family.

Led by Professor Robert Winston, the Genesis Research Trust raises money for the largest UK-based collection of scientists and clinicians who are researching the causes and cures for conditions that affect the health of women and babies. This trust is uniquely based in the building where the scientists carry out their research at the Wolfson and Weston Research Institute for Family Health, on the Hammersmith Campus of Imperial College London.

The objectives of the trust are to provide financial assistance for medical research and teaching in the field of gynaecology, obstetrics and related fields in paediatrics. The trust is organised in order to promote, by all available means, the study of healthy childbearing and diseases of women. Our teaching programme is internationally recognised and the work produced has the highest reputation among academics and researchers. Our courses and symposia are attended by approximately 3,000 full- and part-time students per year.

Advances in the well-being of women and babies can only be achieved by research into the disorders that can affect anyone. Our primary aim is to improve the health of the unborn child and its mother.

The Essential Parent Company

www.essentialparent.com

If you would like more information about our company and the fertility, pregnancy, birth and baby-care online courses we create, please visit our website.